Inspiration, enthusiasm, strength, joy,
and outer supply
come to you in ever-increasing measure
as you depend upon the only Source there is
for your sufficiency.

Myrtle Fillmore

The Handbook

for

Happy Living

by Victoria Morse, Ph.D.

Light Energy Press
Sacramento, California

WWW.VICTORIAMORSE.COM

Publisher's Cataloging
Morse, Victoria
The Handbook for Happy Living / Victoria Morse

Library of Congress Control Number: 2007904645

ISBN: 13 (soft cover) 978-0-9797161-0-2
1. Philosophy 2. Psychology 3. Personal Development

Light Energy Press
Sacramento, California
Printed in U.S.A.

TABLE OF **Contents**

Happiness is like a butterfly,
which when pursued,
Is always just beyond your grasp,
But which,
if you sit down quietly,
may alight upon you.

Nathaniel Hawthorne

Introduction

You must be the change you wish to see in the world.

Mahatma Gandhi

Congratulations on picking up a book with the word *happy* in its title! We all write our own scripts in life, and perhaps we've neglected to pencil in enough mirth. Maybe your choice is to have more fun, but the disasters that seem to take place daily have caused your spirits to sag.

Are you sensitive to the energies around you? Then you need a handbook to help you stay on the happy track. **The Handbook for Happy Living** is a trusty little guide to remind you of what you already know. There's nothing really new here. Proven principles are conveniently gathered in one little volume expressly to make you happy.

You probably think you know who you are. And you picked up this book because *happy* is what you'd like to *be.* Unless you are in deep depression, and I embrace you if you are, you are reasonably happy most of the time, or at least sometimes. If you could extend that *happy* ratio, you probably have the instinctive gut feeling it would enhance your prosperity, your love life, your success with work, family, and friends.

We've learned that we are like radio transmitters, broadcasting our state of mind and emotions to others. If we could broadcast more *happy,* then we would receive in return more *happy* back into our energy fields. What a simple idea to create a more enjoyable life! It's worth taking this valuable little book into your possession, because as you desire to practice its principles, and this becomes a commitment, you will receive the rewards that happiness brings.

Being happy is a decision you choose to make. We are not plopped here in this world with the expectation that everyone will make it right for us. We are born into this time and space because we choose the particular lessons and people that will join us on our road to fulfillment. No one else is to blame for our faulty scriptwriting. With the help of this book, you can choose to be whatever you desire. Rewrite your script if you must. Everything is up to you.

Some people are given difficult circumstances. A wonderful gentleman who was born blind practiced eye exercises every day for hours until little by little he was able to see. The man who defied blindness, Meir Schneider, today has a school in San Francisco. At his seminar his words were: "This is what life handed me, and I have made the best of it." He is genuinely happy helping others by his teaching and example. He exclaims that he never wears glasses, and that yes, he, too, has a driver's license!

You may laugh, but remain compassionate. We never know if another is going through a tragic or stressful situation. Life is full of inequities. Some may be thinking, "You don't know the pain I've been through." "You had both parents," or "You don't know my mother." Many are orphaned, diseased, abused, violated; and still *happiness* is something we can attain a measure of, in spite of circumstances. It's an inside job. It's a life work, but isn't that what life is about?

People come home from war frazzled and broken; they may be maimed, or without limbs. People have seen horrors that are difficult to wipe out of memory. Can they, too, ever find happiness again?

Finding happiness is what this little book is about. We need to grow in forbearance and grace. It's a simple handbook, not psychotherapy. It's a start in the right direction for you to seek out and find the help you need to bring some sparkle back alive. Your happiness is up to you. You decide. You accept where you are and make the decision to capitalize on whatever you've got going for you.

Don't you love the wheelchair olympics! Aren't you in awe of the inspiring foot and mouth painting artists? Sometimes from nothing, people have found a way to serve, inspire, participate and educate to help others overcome obstacles. They work at it. They find joy in it.

Happiness isn't something the world or your mother owes you when you arrive. You may think you are supposed to sit like a baby bird with your beak open. Food and constant entertainment are to be provided to keep you fat and amused. If you reach thirty and still believe you should be getting more, you must take a hard look at what you've been giving out. "What have I to give others?" is a great question.

"What talents can I share?" It's never too late to develop your talents, to learn new skills, or to find your niche. Happy is what you will begin to feel if the path you walk leads you through the chapters and practices outlined in this book. Read on, and enjoy your decision to be happy. Accept your birthright, and the rewards of a life filled with peace and joy.

Happiness consists of being and doing good.

Mary Baker Eddy

If you want happiness for an hour - take a nap

If you want happiness for a day - go fishing

If you want happiness for a month - get married

If you want happiness for a year - inherit a fortune

If you want happiness for a lifetime - help someone else

Chinese Proverb

Live simply and be content
with innocent pleasures...

I know longer try to compel anything.
I have come to understand within my own consciousness
A reason for everything that happens to me,
or ever will.
And I do not blame people or conditions anymore,
Or blame myself, for this is a matter of consciousness;
Instead, I try to provide a greater consciousness.

Ernest Holmes

Live Simply

When you are content to be simply yourself and don't compare or compete, everybody will respect you.

Lao Tzu

You don't have to live like a monk. But it wouldn't hurt. Once I cleaned out everything and thought I should try living out of one suitcase. I was to house-sit so this was the perfect opportunity to see if I was up to the dare. I put basic things in storage, as this was to be a five month trial where I would be staying in three different homes for vacationing friends. It wasn't easy for someone who loves clothes and shoes, but it was the best thing I ever did!

Paring down gives you the chance to value what is truly important to you. Years ago when I lived near a river which was to overflow its banks during a flood, the thought of my belongings being wiped out set me to choices I could put in my car and drive to the high ground of a friend's. The river did not overflow, but I could sleep that night, and have never forgotten what I chose to take with me. Each might select differently what is most valuable. I took important papers, my jewelry box, other meaningful items, but most of all I wanted the family pictures.

We don't need all the stuff we accumulate. It takes continual clearing out to keep our energies free for creative endeavors. Beautiful mementos of our remembered loved ones have their place. Artistic furnishings and cherished reminders of home and comfort can be individualized to meet the families' needs - but "happy" isn't clutter!

We've heard that less is better. If you want to keep things simple, this is true. Encumbrance with excesses can cause energy drain and stress. Would you like me to tell you an easy way to unload? Order a dumpster delivered to your driveway. That's what a fellow I know did when a family member passed. To clean everything out, he gave himself two weeks to empty house and garage for painting and putting it on the market.

If you don't want to do something this drastic, take one room at a time and dispose of useless or superfluous stuff by taking it to The Salvation Army. Items you haven't used, or clothes you haven't worn in a year are sapping your energy space where new ideas and joys are born. Free up and let go the past so that freshness and newness can bring in *happy* vibes.

Entanglements, enmeshments that drain your peace of mind and cause you worry or stress must also go. You say your husband or wife is the packrat. You say your children or work leave your life anything but simple. It's up to you to simplify. Your vibrations on overload will attract more overload. That's why it is a MUST that you begin the simplification process now. It starts with cleaning out the clutter!

That done, you'll have renewed energy. Get rid of books, CD's, and household items that can be circulated for someone else's good. Circulation is not stagnant but flowing. Get into the flow of circulating good and you will find happiness revolving back to you with less stress and simple living.

Simple living and Zen are not easy. It takes effort to attain nothingness. And then what do you have?

A Jewish Buddhist

A Promise in March

I open myself as wide
As this sky and these fields
To your holy presence.
As the new buds and blossoms hold promise
Of beauty and fragrance,
So your presence in me
Holds promise of wondrous good.
I do not doubt in the face of the March sky.
Clouds pass and dissipate.
Patches of blue confirm that
The vault of heaven is untouched!

In the bleakness of any of life's experiences,
A deep assurance of eternity
Holds me steady and strong.
I spring forth into newness of life!

I do not doubt in the face of the March sky!

Dorothy Pierson

Whenever I decide something with kindness,
I mostly make the right decision.

Speak Kindly

We can be spacious yet full of loving kindness; full of compassion, yet serene. Live like the strings of a fine instrument - not too taut but not too loose.

The Buddha

Speak the truth, but speak it palatably.

Sanskrit Proverb

It's so easy to judge another. As you think, so you get. What you say about another you are implying about yourself. Your words are so important because your subconscious acts them out on you, not the other person.

When one speaks kindly it will be passed along, generating more kindness in its transmission. When someone is fighting a hard battle, one thoughtful word can change his experience and uplift his day. If we could stay level enough to rain our kindness equally on everyone, wouldn't we have arrived at a happy state of serenity? It's worth working toward.

Sometimes parents find it easy to be civil and friendly to others and lose it when it comes to their own children. Overworked mothers, heedless of the damage that can be inflicted on their child's esteem, have been heard giving tongue lashings they are later ashamed took place. No one wants to be at wit's end. We want to be happy, to feel balanced, to speak kindly and appropriately.

Get enough sleep. Perhaps a vitamin supplement such as B vitamins and magnesium would aid the nervous system. If you have addictions, those must go. You will have to find a blood cleanser to remove toxins from the body. Happiness is hard to come by if you are not clean inside and out.

It may be difficult to speak kindly if it has not been given to you as a child. Again, the decision to speak kindly can be learned. Our words shape our lives and bring full circle the vibrations we project. This can't be emphasized enough! Never argue. Nobody wins.

We function like transmitters. The words and frequencies we emit from our mouths find their way back into our lives. Listening to endless diatribes of rap, mindless noise, television or computer conundrum doesn't lead to happiness, but unfortunately to more of the same.

If we want joy, then we must speak of the joy and beauty around us. The "good" we focus on extends a wave-length; and a channel has been created to return "good" back to us. Speak kindly of others and judge not. You cannot possibly know the sadness or difficulties another has gone through.

I was driving on a busy boulevard when the car in front of me was weaving and slowing, As I tried to pass, he veered back into the passing lane. With signs of disgust, I muttered a few words, which I soon had to eat. As I finally managed to get around him, I looked his direction and saw a prominent patch bandaged over his left eye. I was humbled, and softly vowed to drive with more compassionate understanding. My words had been wrongly directed and I was the one suffering humiliation from uttering them.

Be flexible enough to give a listening ear to hear where others are coming from, and not just what they're saying or how they are acting. This is especially true if they are swearing or screaming. "Peace Be Still" can surely be felt when one speaks kindly.

Remember that silence is sometimes the best answer.
The Dalai Lama

Peace

Peace flows through my heart, and blows through
me as a zephyr.
Peace fills me like a fragrance.
Peace runs through me like rays.
Peace stabs the heart of noise and worries.
Peace burns through my disquietude.
Peace, like a globe of fire, expands and fills
my omnipresence.
Peace, like an ocean, rolls on in all space.
Peace, like red blood, vitalizes the veins of
my thoughts.
Peace like a boundless aureole, encircles my
body of infinity.
Peace-flames blow through the pores of my
flesh, and through all space.
The perfume of peace flows over the gardens
of blossoms.
The wine of peace runs perpetually through
the wine press of all hearts.
Peace is the breath of stones, stars, and
sages.
Peace is the ambrosial wine of Spirit flowing
from the cask of silence,
Which I quaff with my countless mouths of
atoms.

Paramahansa Yogananda

For the Children:

A Happy Heart

(Tune of Jimmy Cracks Corn and I Don't Care)

Look at me
I have a Happy Heart.
You can see
I have a Happy Heart.
Joy within me
Makes all cares depart
For I have a Happy Heart.

Listen to me
It's my Happy Heart
Singing through me
It's my Happy Heart
Blues and sadness
Never get a start
For I have a Happy Heart!

Bonnie Beam

If You're Happy and You Know It

(Tune of She'll be Comin' 'Round the Mountain)

If you're happy and you know it, clap your hands,
If you're happy and you know it, clap your hands,
If you're happy and you know it, then your face will surely show it,
If you're happy and you know it, clap your hands!
(2) stamp your feet
(3) say amen

I Need a Friend

I need a friend, I need a pal,
Someone to talk to
Someone right now.
I feel alone, but if I have you
My dreams of friendship
Might really come true.

Friends are so important
'Cause we need someone to care,
Someone in our corner
When we thought no one was there;
One to share our triumphs with
As well as our despair,
We need friends there.

I need a friend, do they need me?
Maybe they're lonely
And I just can't see.
If I be the kind of friend
That I need
My dreams of friendship
Might really succeed.

Friends are so important
'Cause without 'em it's no fun.
Friends to joke and laugh with
Make your life a happy one.
A friend to throw an arm around
To hug when there's a tear,
We need friends near.

I'm glad my friends are here!

Victoria Morse

The Subject Tonight is Love

The subject tonight is Love

And for tomorrow night as well,

As a matter of fact

I know of no better topic

For us to discuss

Until we all

Die!

Hafitz

The Happy Virus

I caught the happy virus last night

When I was out singing beneath the stars.

It is remarkably contagious -

So kiss me.

Hafitz

Love Generously

The beginning of love is to let those we love be perfectly themselves, and not to twist them to fit our own image. Otherwise we love only the reflection of ourselves we find in them.

Thomas Merton

Who can define love? At the core of our desires are we not one? More than any other single thing, don't we all want acceptance? Accept folks for who they are, generously, without reticence. This is not to say condone unacceptable behavior. Rather, look into the soul and discard personal sense. "My" life, my education, my health, wealth, intelligence can sometimes get in the way of seeing another in a loving light, or seeing them at all!

I was taught to ignore children because I was ignored. This is no excuse! It is something I work on, noticing and responding to people, no matter what age child they are. We must step out of ourselves and into the other fellow's shoes in acknowledging or greeting them.

With compassion we can look for the good in every being. We're going to extend to others as we would have them extend to us; treat others as we would like to be treated. Ask yourself, "How can I love more?" Make the request of your higher power, "Teach me to love," and you will undoubtedly be provided with ample opportunities.

I remember when I was a busy student and had to shop late after a class. It was after 10:30 at night and I pulled into the driveway and opened the trunk. I saw a shadow pass and turned quickly to lock the gates behind me before the dogs would come bounding up. As I pulled one side of the chain link gate closed, reaching for the other side to hand clasp the lock around, a tall figure loomed up three feet from me. I said in a strong voice of conviction, "Watch out for the dogs! I don't want them to hurt you." The man cowered and said, "How big are those dogs?" "Don't worry," I said. "I'm locking this gate so they won't get you." Up lumbered my two harmless pets, one, big enough in the shadows to look protective, and the small one, *yippy* enough to make noise. The man slipped away, saying "Thanks," and muttering, "I don't want those dogs to get me."

The man could have easily pulled the gate out of my hands, but I had the presence of mind to do and say what was best for all concerned. *The Presence* is what we're after. When we practice "presence of mind," we know what to do and when to do it. I won't say my knees didn't buckle a bit afterward when I brought the groceries into the house. Something had come over me in a time of need, which I knew was greater than my *personal* self. It really blessed us both. I felt a kinship with that man when he said, "Thanks." I've known since then that I can look beyond the appearance, and listen for the guidance to say and do what is appropriate for the circumstance. I can value human dignity, and I can love generously.

Life may not be as happy for some without sex, so let's broach the subject here. When you love generously, don't let that give you license to have sex promiscuously. Love is a matter of the heart, and deeply intertwined with the emotions. If entered into lightly, the results can only be less than real love, and perhaps heartbreaking, even devastating for one or both parties.

Hold sacred the sanctity of your union, and you will find life richer with generous love as you nurture your growth together. If sex becomes a matter of convenience, both parties lose. Keep it sweet. Keep it fed mutually by loving consideration and mutual response. When there are children, the demands for generosity are far greater. The patience, perseverance, principled decisions with realistic expectations are character-building, to say the least. Let love reign in every household. Stand firm in the foundation you build, disciplined with respect and love.

Always remember that someone cutting you off in traffic may be the mother of four who just worked nine hours and is going to school evenings. Or the young lane-swapping speedster who is taking school exams, is worried about his student loans for next year, and has just been jilted by his girlfriend. Have mercy on the street people asking for money. There, but for the grace of God, go I.

Show compassion on a slow moving person ahead of you, who may have just learned the worst after a biopsy. Scary looking bums, or those abusive and aggressive, may be slaves to addictions that we cannot imagine. We don't know another's pain. We can appreciate empathy. The greatest gift we will ever possess is love.

Everywhere we look people with crying needs are seeking love, understanding, and compassion. Every day's mail contains solicitations to help the starving children, to feed and clothe destitute families, to create shelter and stability for those wiped out by famine or flood. Nowhere do we find a lack of charities to love generously. If you do not feel loved, then the quickest antidote is to give to others in greater need than yourself.

The way to love is the way of oneness; no personal sense, no human will, no desire, but to let life live through you as love!

I do not fear tomorrow for I have seen yesterday and I love today.

William Allen White

It is love that brings happiness to people.
It is love that gives joy to happiness. Rumi

Enough Love

There is no difficulty that enough love will not conquer;
No disease that enough love will not heal;
No door that enough love will not open;
No gulf that enough love will not bridge;
No wall that enough love will not throw down;
No sin that enough love will not redeem.
It makes no difference how deeply seated may be the trouble,
How hopeless the outlook,
How muddled the tangle,
How great the mistake;
A sufficient realization of love will dissolve it all.
If only you could love enough, you would be the happiest and most powerful being in the world.

Emmet Fox

Care Deeply

Love first ourselves; love then our neighbors, and our neighbors as ourselves. That's true love and peace, and it will end wars.

We each set in motion the commotion in our lives, or we set in motion love and peace.

Melanie A. Sprague

How do you establish your day first thing in the morning? Recognize that you are included in a joyful creation and you hold within you everything you need to fulfill your day. You can decide to be happy about *everything*, even if it's raining outside! Free your mind from worries declaring, "I am filled with right ideas from my Source. I know what to do and how to do it." Sit up in bed and meditate for at least two minutes before getting started with your day.

Identify yourself with the Presence within. Your "true self" will shine today and supersede any negative degradation. Then, accept as fact that your day is established in good work and right activity. Let nothing dampen your spirit or pull you down. If you see anything unlovely in your family, change your view. As you see it, so be it. You want to be a vibrating match with your Source drawing to you the good you are holding in consciousness. Lift your spirits to joy. Fake it till you make it.

Every person is surrounded by an energy field which broadcasts the kind of emotions experienced. If deep in the subconscious there is fear, resentment, animosity, or some unresolved hurt, let it go through breathing and meditation. You must care deeply about yourself first! You must let go the old patterns and embark on the new way of looking at yourself. Cleanse the old patterns with a positive outlook. Look from the other side of the coin. See differently. Stay out of doubt, insecurity, or dysfunctional relationships by focusing on that which you would like to experience. What you fill your mind with, what you focus on, becomes your reality. So dare to dream the "good" into your day.

Desire, decide, and DO whatever it takes to accomplish your day's goals. At the end of the day when you look back at what you have achieved, you are inspired to make attainable goals every day, and then goals for a year, or for five years!

There is one major goal I believe worth attaining. It is to "Know Thyself." It's a one man show, and only you can make it happen. It takes quiet introspection. It takes communion with your inner being, and for that one needs some silence and alone time on occasion. Find moments to be still. Entertain your own thoughts and record them in a journal if you wish. You and your ideas bring a valuable contribution to the whole scheme of things. That's why you are here on the planet. You are to offer your talent in a beneficial way. Put to use your good qualities.

Perhaps I have the talent for being calm in a tense situation. I was working for a housing agency in an office at one of the sites. My boss was nowhere to be found when I heard a blood-curdling scream coming from the laundry room two doors down. I headed that direction. Entering as if it was my duty, I found a man trying to strangle his wife. Two very frightened children about eight and four years old stood frozen with eyes wide. Drawing on the Presence, I put my hands on my hips and said, "There is entirely too much noise going on here!" "We can't work in this clamor!" "You'll have to be quiet," I said.

A wild-eyed man took his hands from the shrieking woman's throat and started towards me. "Are you going to interfere here?" he said, both hands up ready to take me on next. I planted my feet and stared him right in the eyes.

What occurred then was something I'll never forget. I saw the child in his wild eyes. For a moment they were the eyes of a four-year-old. They had glared at me, bloodshot; then softened. He dropped his hands and looked down. Then his wife let out another shriek, and he lunged back for her throat. I commanded a "Hush!" to her that stilled her in mid-scream.

The man dropped his hands, and stooped to pick up his little boy to hold him in his arms. He appeared from that point on to be sober and docile. The police arrived, I went back to my office, and that was the end of it.

When you care deeply, you will do what is yours to do. Not all of us are given the same tasks. We have different purposes, but you will know when it is in your capacity to act or be a spokesperson for peace, kindness, or good work. You have to live in the NOW, always ready from your "first thing in the morning" preparation.

The greatest secret to happiness is to live consciously with intention. Make it your intention to care deeply. Be passionate about what you love, and you will develop capabilities that may surprise you. Who knew that as a young woman I would stand fearless in a life-threatening situation? Wisdom prevails when your motive is compassion. Fear in catastrophic confrontation is out of the question. We know not in advance how to handle everything that comes up, so we must trust *The Presence* in the moment. Its intuitive guidance will direct our manner and actions. If words are needed, they will come to mind.

At commencement time politicians, activists, and prominent personalities are invited to address graduates at the different colleges. Sage and stirring advice is selected with care. From Katie Couric, TV journalist speaking at Williams College, she touched on the fact that today's upward mobility requires constant availability. She said that between the ages of 18 and 40, the average American holds 10 different jobs. This was Couric's counsel: "No matter how much potential you think you have, a little humility will serve you well - and help you focus on doing your best in the job you've got, rather than plotting to get the job you think you deserve."

Actress Marlee Matlin shared insights the same year at Wilkes University: "As a woman growing up deaf, who wanted to be an actress, despite what others may have thought was possible, I know firsthand what wonder there is if we consider what is possible. And I know the same is true for you...Ó "Along the way, don't forget to volunteer, to love, to laugh, pay your taxes, but most of all, never forget to listen. Listen to your hearts."

Every day of your life you deposit happy moments into a bank account. On dark days, you can draw on a happy memory. Deposit lots of joy, laughter, good deeds, caring and thoughtfulness into your account and you will be rich! These deposits will pay dividends your life through.

We all care deeply for those wounded, ill, oppressed, or imprisoned. You will be motivated by your inner purpose to help others in your individual way. Follow through on your leadings. Listen to your guidance, and when you do, you will begin to experience a soul satisfaction and happiness that brings contentment like nothing else can.

The greatest gift we can give each other is love. It's free, so start now. Give a smile, give a hug. Be a little frisky. Go ahead, set it in motion. Live love!

Melanie A. Sprague

Spreading Divine Joy

Beginning with early dawn each day, I will radiate joy to everyone I meet. I will be mental sunshine for all who cross my path. I will burn candles of smiles in the bosoms of the joyless. Before the unfading light of my cheer, darkness will take flight.

Let my love spread its laughter in all hearts, in every person belonging to every race. Let my love rest in the hearts of flowers, of animals, and of little specs of stardust.

I will try to be happy under all circumstances. I will make up my mind to be happy within myself right now, where I am today.

Let my soul smile through my heart and let my heart smile through my eyes, that I may scatter Thy rich smiles in sad hearts.

Paramahansa Yogananda

For you, from a sister...

Healthy, Wealthy and Wise

Many things happen as years pass
But truly you remain the same,
Never compromising your faith
Though you are deserving of fame.

The lovely child you were back then
You have brought with you to this time,
Adding grace, intelligence, fun
And talent. You are at your prime.

Never question your place in life;
You are living it every day.
It is "now" that counts, not the next,
As you follow your ordained way.

The love you feel, the joy you give
Comes back to you time and again.
Don't look for them in the outward things;
They are there when you look within.

I stand by you observing truths,
As I know they belong to you.
I send you love and joy and mirth,
As I know for me, you do, too.

I cannot give to you your wealth;
Your health is of my caring.
I cannot bring you your wisdom;
Your Source supports your bearing.

As a new year starts afresh for you
Remember, money never buys
The treasures you have brought to earth.
You came Healthy, Wealthy and Wise.

Marilyn Outerbridge

Spend Wisely

...an't buy you happiness.
...ring you a more pleasant
... misery.

Spike Milligan

Owe no one anything, except to love one another...

Romans 13:8

Pay off your credit cards every month and spend wisely. You may like looking prosperous and enjoy shopping, but you are not staying in harmony with your best interests if you are a spendthrift. You want to work toward financial freedom. You want to owe no one so that you are fully free to care deeply and love generously. Being heavily in debt is an energy drain that places enormous stress on your body and your relationships.

When finances are not healthy, money is not what's the matter. It's limited thinking, a belief in separation from your Source. Close the gap of separation by thinking and spending in terms of oneness with the kind of abundance you truly value. All good is ours by perceiving the amazing gifts we already possess. Fresh air, sunshine, those who love us, and the ability to love them back - that's the gift. That's a wealth to share until we can actually give from our overflow to charities.

Get off what you don't like about your job and onto the benefits of what you *do* have. Applying the happy living principle of living within your means, you can be thankful for where you work at the moment. Do your best, perform a service, and it can bring you into your next work.

A young woman who intensely disliked her job as a clerk decided to change her attitude. She would dress impeccably to add professionalism, and show respect for her customers. She laid out her clothes the night before, making certain they were fresh and unwrinkled. She was careful with hygiene, selected an appropriate hair style, and generally dressed for success. She felt better about herself, which was apparent in her courteous helpful service. It wasn't long before one of her customers noticed her demeanor and invited her to work at his prosperous insurance firm. It was a dream job for her in an atmosphere where upward mobility was possible.

We must do our best, give our best, be our best. Higher levels of desire to serve well evolve us to the place where we find appreciation and can grow.

Financial freedom isn't something out there somewhere meant for someone else. It takes your desire and focus. It's work, but it's worth staying with it for the long haul. Right where you are is what you have created. In your own back yard your "diamond in the rough" is buried. It's up to you to uncover and polish every facet of yourself - to magnify and share your gifts so they may bring in your remuneration.

You are *always* paid for what you do. No work goes unrewarded, even if it appears to be thankless at the time. Remember that little verse? *I do wonderful work in a wonderful way; with wonderful people for wonderful pay.*

Whatever you think and speak about, you get more of it. Abundance Is! If it's a truth principle, it operates unspent. You may use it over and over again and watch the truth principle operate in your life. Do what you must, and be "happy" doing it. Choosing to be happy is the first step on the path to financial freedom where your debts will be paid.

It's an energy drag when you are in debt and it can divide the family. Work toward financial freedom where less is more, and you are unencumbered with burdens. Try not using a charge card and pay cash. Watch your savings grow! If you have addictions, gambling debts, or are over your head with bills, now is the time to face up to it and stop the spiral.

An acquaintance of mine had a series of bad turns. Her husband had overspent stocking a hardware store that went belly-up within a year. He couldn't face the failure, and moved out of town leaving her with two young children to pick up the pieces. She used every resource she had to pay off the debts. Wisely, she called the creditors and worked out specific ways to pay them back. It took some years, but this woman is happy, fulfilled, and living a prosperous life today.

When the real estate market dropped in 1990, I had just put everything I owned, including an inheritance from my deceased father, into a house which dropped in value so drastically I was forced to let it be repossessed. I tried sending in payments which were returned. Valiantly I looked for a buyer, but it was no go. The market had turned so sour that putting any more money in was like pouring water down the drain. All I could do was hold my head up, sell everything to neighbors and friends, and rent a room in someone's home. A backyard spa I had put in under a little gazebo I doggedly sold to a neighbor. That paid for my move. Wiped out in every way, I declared vehemently, "There's more where that came from."

I did not feel destitute, and this I believe, is the secret. I felt triumphant that I did have a plan. I could let go of "stuff," and hold on to my dignity while moving into two rooms as a renter. I was allowed to store some items in the garage for which I was deeply grateful.

A new surge of energy swept through my life. I had to let go first; then work my way toward a newly opening vista.

Everybody wants to be financially secure. What I had hoped was going to be a sound investment did not turn out that way. Most people are afraid of the future and a lack of financial stability. Allay this fear! Don't put all your eggs into one basket. The best way to get ahead is to become a business owner doing duplicatable direct selling. For a very low start up fee my nutrition company helps me earn passive income while I still keep a day job. Over the years this will build momentum. I love working toward financial freedom by just sharing the products I use myself. I will never be out of work, but will always keep actively occupied and useful. Several gentlemen I know have continued going to their offices well into their 80's; and one is teaching seminars at 92.

Open the channels of your mind to lay claim to your prosperity. It's always already within you. Live within your means and pay your bills on time. As you listen to your inner voice, you will be guided to take the right steps with self assurance that you are worthy to receive your good today - and each day that you tune in to your higher "happy" being.

The more joy we have, the more nearly perfect we are.

Spinosa

Yesterday is a cancelled check;
Tomorrow is a promissory note;
Today is the only cash you have –
So spend it wisely.

Kay Lyon

Share in Relationships

By all means, marry. If you get a good wife, you'll become happy; if you get a bad one, you'll become a philosopher. Socrates

It is cowardice to perceive what is right but not to do it. Confucius

It is a recorded fact that most men live longer being married; and for women, those single are seeing an increase in longevity. With such a dichotomy it's no wonder that relational changes are taking place that allow more space for individuals to grow. This can't help but be a good thing, no matter what lifestyle you choose.

Children should be our first priority. They are the joy of today and the future. The greatest emphasis placed on their healthy growth, education and strength of character can promote family happiness and relationship delight. Giving of yourself creates soul satisfaction. Our children need listening ears, wise counsel, and peaceful attendance. Share with them, love them, and listen. In so doing, you will nurture a communication with your own inner child that can also benefit from the relationship. We need one another to show an interest in our endeavors or unfoldments. How, but by sharing, can we communicate happy life experiences?

No one is in charge of your happiness but you. If you are going to put your children in charge of making decisions before they are six, don't be surprised if they don't choose oatmeal or broccoli. Stubborn and resistant children can make life unhappy at times, but you have trained them. Teach right choices and help them decide wisely. Their self esteem grows when there is mutual agreement, even when in certain instances, you must overrule their immature judgment. Your children learn from your decisions and your actions much more than from your talk. With love as your motive they will feel it.

Voicing praise or appreciation is always welcome when valid. Everyone wants to be loved and respected. If you are going to point a finger, or make the other person wrong, that's the start of a war. Don't do it. Try to see where they're coming from. You don't have to win every argument. You can agree to disagree. But if the other is trying to rub you out, take the hint and take a hike. It's simple to say, "Treat others as you would be treated." Now do that! Include yourself. There's the challenge.

Trust is a huge factor in relationship harmony. If you can recognize your gut feeling as a reliable moral compass, this will aid you in selecting your partner, and in maintaining friendships. If your word is good, if you live up to your promises, if you follow through, how happy are those around you! They can relax with faith in your integrity. You can fulfill yourself only if you are trustworthy and honest in your actions and dealings with others.

If you are in a relationship based on convenience which is not a harmonious match, then you must refine your desires and qualities to lift your consciousness. Work on yourself - not the other guy. Life is appearing to you the way you see it. You may need to change your view. For changes to take place, you must love where you are at the moment. It's no good hating anyone or anything. Life it too short to harm yourself that severely.

Find the good in everything and every one and give thanks for it. It's the only way to draw more good to yourself. Your vibrations will draw more of what you are feeling, so keep your words in sync with your feelings and watch what transpires. Sound simple? It's a life work we must be about doing.

There were two clients who came to me asking why they couldn't bear children. One decided to adopt, the other tried invitro-fertilization and had a second child a year later. Another couple had twins from the fertilization process. All are delighted with their precious progeny.

A dear friend who had adopted two, lost the talented elder one at age twenty three. How must his brother have felt who nursed him in rehab for two years? He and the parents can only make peace knowing they did their best.

Two others in our neighborhood who it seemed had everything to live for, took their own lives before age thirty. This sad loss must be addressed. We gain nothing by going elsewhere to solve our problems. Drugs and suicide are not the answer. It is all too easy to overdose on anti-depressants. Young people who have unrealistic expectations, or feel lovelorn or forgotten must know that this earth plane is where all the lessons are learned.

Those who move on before completing them will return at some point to finish their assignments. It's a simple explanation for why I believe in reincarnation. We each have certain purposes to fulfill, and we may as well get at it. The more we procrastinate, the more life-times we go through to do our job right. If possible, learn to do it right from the start.

A woman I know was married three years when her husband wanted another child. He was so adamant that he withheld sex. She had two sons from a prior marriage and an adorable little girl from the marriage with him. She was offered an editorship of a local newspaper, but felt she must decline as the little girl was only two. Her mother had just died and she was also in grief. She simply could not agree to having a fourth child, as in her saddened state she felt she would die in childbirth. When her young daughter turned four, she filed for divorce. She deeply wanted to fulfill her purpose, and did not regret the decision.

If you don't know your purpose - and we all have one - it's best to find out what you love and where you shine early on. It's okay to refine it as you go along. You have a talent that must be shared, and sometimes it's more winsomely accomplished in partnerships. That's why our relationships should be given "divine" status. What we accomplish together may become magnificent! Or work on your own, but find support networks.

Your spouse should add to your expertise rather that demote or deflate your purpose. Find partners and friends that build you up rather than denigrate your efforts. This goes for family as well. If your true purpose runs at odds with your family, church, or synagogue's values, here is where you must make decisions that will enhance your own peace of mind. You cannot live at cross-purposes with yourself and be happy. Only you know where you must draw lines and boundaries, and take your stand for being true to the guidance of your higher power.

Regarding marriage, I found I needed more alone time and opted for the single life for fifteen years. I so wanted the right *"one,"* but dedicated myself to fulfilling everything I possibly desired, practicing public speaking through Toastmasters International, making my jazz vocal CD, taking music. I wanted to teach dance and did. I directed a small choir and provided choreography for a dozen performers. I gained credentials in virtually all of the healing arts and worked from my office in a medical building to successfully serve a burgeoning clientele. Immersed in work, I wasn't actively *"looking"* to date.

Finally, a fellow I've known for twelve years came in to where I was working part-time and said, "We should go out to dinner." People have always said it's when you're not looking that you find what works compatibly.

I still keep my own apartment. My lifestyle of meditation and writing requires living alone for now. My wonderful partner enjoys his house and garage, and we're both happy. I can't say enough about giving each other leeway to be free as individuals with time to be creative.

One of my clients was lamenting her lack of dates. She took a class in something that interested her and struck up a conversation with a man in the class. As far as I know they are still together. You can be best friends, married or not. Good friends are like stars. You don't always see them, but you know they are always there. Embrace folks into your life and be blessed.

Honor and adore your pets, and savor your long-time friendships. Be always open to new acquaintances joining your relationship circle. For most men, marriage gives them greater satisfaction and health. Women have lamented to me that their husbands don't give them breathing space and time alone. They may want to write a poem, gentlemen!

Here are the words of a song I wrote for a play by the same title:

Marriage Hasn't Worked for Me

People everywhere walking hand in hand
Sharing a heart of serenity;
Laughing, smiling at each other's glance,
But marriage hasn't worked for me.

What must I do to be in the crowd
Of happy folks who've found the one they love?
Why does my heart want to cry out loud?
Bring me the one that I'm dreamin' of.

I've searched near and far, now I know it's true
If marriage hasn't worked
Take the inside view.
I'll work for IT; make the vow to commit,
I'm going to give it a hundred and ten percent!

I want it to be; will WORK FOR IT 'til I see
That marriage finally works for me.

Victoria Morse

Seek Spiritual Practices

I saw Eternity the other night
Like a great ring of pure and endless light.
Henry Vaughan

Before you take another step, step back into yourself.
If you can govern yourself and be your own master,
yours is the whole wide world and everything within it.
Paul Fleming

There is a divinity in all humankind. You are beloved souls. Your spark of life inside connects you to your Source and every living thing. You are an integral and necessary part of the universal design. To become more fully aware of your place and purpose is your earth mission. It is to do your best and to be happy!

The resistance to this is terrific. Everything tries to pull you down and squash out the joy. Don't allow it. It is a decision for you to smile. It is a decision for you to reclaim your childlike innocence and start new each day with pure motives. Commune with your Higher Being upon waking each morning. Start fresh before you rise, mentally declaring that you are worthy of respect and value. Honor yourself by allowing a few moments of silent connection with your holy innermost being. Take deep breaths until you find peace and harmony within, and see peace and harmony manifesting in your day.

You will find this such a benefit to your achievements that you will not want to miss your quiet meditation time each morning. The one thing we all have in common is a spiritual impulse. We know there is something higher, better, that will enlighten and enoble us. Just the opposite from dragging us down, this spiritual impulse lifts us to raise our sights above the material picture. Sometimes we're forced to view something better than the appearance presenting itself at the moment. That's a way to move through it and go on. We can't stay stuck in the past and expect to move forward as if putting on the gas and the brakes at the same time. Let go. Don't stay on it. Reach for the spiritual insight. Learn from mistakes and stay with your higher consciousness. Always go for the good. Refuse to wallow in garbage or allow it into your experience.

At the time my sister passed away I became so angry. She lived in another state and I couldn't see that her condition was more serious than she had let on. It was such a shock to learn she expired from an enlarged heart. I was overwhelmed with grief and could only handle the injustice of it through prayer and meditation. No other way could I be consoled. The anger persisted, and to this day, over ten years later, I still resort to peaceful meditation whenever I think of her special sweetness.

If you want to, you can erase your past in an instant. Look at your present qualities. Jot down the best of yourself, and focus on that. Focus on the person you desire to be. Then claim your present acknowledgement and drop the old movie. You've as much ability to do this as you desire. Just as you would change the channels on a remote, prove for yourself it's that easy to make a switch from the old pattern.

No one can find out their own soul's desire by following a particular teaching and obeying its rules and regulations. You must quietly search within to discover your unique purpose. As you perform daily what is yours to do, the evolution takes place and you become more certain what work will teach you along your path. We live to learn.

If you have a church, synagogue, or a self help group, how wonderful that you have support, and a place to be of service to others. Your spiritual practices are enhanced when you are also there to uplift others. Give of yourself. Be a listening friend when needed.

A walking meditation can give a great low-impact, cardio workout. The focus is on movement while being mindful of things outside yourself. You can enjoy the sights and sounds of nature and feel the sun or wind while being intensely aware of your body. Note each step and how your feet, legs and ankles are involved with your steps. Shift your balance and let your arms hang naturally, allowing your eyes to softly focus several feet in front of you. Try a short 20 minute walking meditation and then imagine being able to meditate while walking across the parking lot to your office.

Prayer is preferred by some. It doesn't need to be petition. Asking for what is already within you is of no avail. You wouldn't pray for light when all you have to do is lift the window shade or flip the light switch. Be still and let the listening ear have precedence. In meditation it's the release of mind chatter for quiet surrender to peace. Eyes closed, the ego loses itself to oneness with Source energy. The soul becomes satisfied in this quiet sanctuary, and a sweet refreshing connection has been made.

Yoga can also help you make this connection. Perhaps with soft music do some stretches and yoga moves. After energization exercises, you may want to meditate in front of your altar. It can be a sacred area in your home where you have pictures, a rosary, a crystal or a favorite rock; a candle, a feather, or something meaningful to your spiritual side. When sitting before your altar, come into a meditative state breathing in love into the abdomen. Breathe out toxins. Take in peace deep to your depths, and exhale stress. Inhale joy and exhale, until only well-being remains. One of my teachers likes to wear a shawl over her head in meditation to help her go within. She feels safely nestled from the world.

Yoga has gained so much popularity in the West by bringing together the union of mind, body, and breath into one practice. Hatha yoga, the standing practice in positions called asanas, can benefit the circulation and bring flexibility and strength to the spine and limbs. Poses are done in connection with breath work which result in a calm focused mind. More energy is produced as the body is stretched and strengthened for a sense of integration and well-being.

Often at the beginning, or at the end of a yoga class, time is given for introspection and meditation which helps the student attune to their higher nature. Over time, with regular practice of yoga, comes a sense of confidence and peaceful life-mastery. For some, balance and a spiritual centeredness are definitive rewards.

Cherished deep refreshment can be found in your spiritual practices. Perhaps, for you, it is an inspiring piece of music. When my daughter was expecting, I gave her a Baby Bach CD. I wanted the new-born to come in with peaceful classics. They say classical compositions help to relieve stress. I tried an experiment playing rock and jazz constantly for a week, and my plants died! I love jazz! I now find times to alternate my music with *Mozart* and The *Best of Tchaikovsky*, as well as fun "big band" or Dixieland.

For quiet relaxation, visit or visualize a favorite spot in nature; the ocean, a river waterfall, or perhaps a mountain path with a view in the forest. Let your soul be restored, and you mind swept clean from worries by yielding time in your day for the contemplation of peace. You'll be happy you did!

Create in me a clean heart; ... and renew a right spirit within me.

Psalms 51: 10

Happiness Radiates

Keep your desires turned back within.
Be patient.
Allow the fulfillment to come to you.
Gently resist the temptation to chase your dreams out in the world.
Pursue them in your heart until they disappear into the Self,
and leave them there.
It may take a little self-discipline.

Be simple, be kind, stay rested.
Attend to your inner health and happiness.

Happiness radiates like the fragrance from a flower,
and draws all good things to you.
Allow your love to nourish yourself as well as others.
Do not strain after your needs in life.
It is sufficient to be quietly alert and aware.
Then in this way life proceeds more
naturally and effortlessly.

Maharishi

Born to Soar

We were not put here on earth to worry,
To fret and doubt to hurry and scurry;
Like happy and trusting birds on the wing,
We were born to soar...and joyfully sing!

William Arthur Ward

A Happy Home Recipe

4 cups of love
2 cups of loyalty
3 cups of forgiveness
1 cup of friendship
5 spoons of hope
2 spoons of tenderness
4 quarts of faith
1 barrel of laughter

Take love and loyalty, mix it thoroughly with faith. Blend it with tenderness, kindness and understanding. Add friendship and hope; sprinkle abundantly with laughter. Bake it with sunshine, Serve daily with generous helpings.

Hone Up on Health and Fitness

People through finding something beautiful
Think something else unbeautiful,
Through finding one man fit
Judge another unfit. Lao Tzu

All things in nature are in balance. Lao Tzu

A man rushed into a busy doctor's office and shouted "Doctor, I think I'm shrinking!" The doctor calmly responded, "Now settle down. You'll just have to be a little patient." How many of you want to be a little patient? Most of us want things larger than life, and yesterday. We frantically search for who or what outside of ourselves can make us well, happy and rich. We want to be secure. We believe if we hold onto enough property, stuff, and weight, that will ensure sustaining a reliable place for us. We wouldn't want to disappear any more than we want to be a little patient.

Your health is your greatest wealth. Being fit without aches or pains is a goal you can strive toward no matter your age. It first takes your desire; then your dedication to follow through with action.

A client of mine said he grew up never being happy. He was afraid of everything and withdrew from people and activities. His family life was good and his brothers and sister seemed normal, but he said he often hid in the closet or behind the couch with fears, quite unhappy.

After working with him, he disclosed his undeniable sweet tooth. I asked if he was given sweets to placate his fears when he was a child. He said he insisted that everything he ate must be sweet. His mother indulged his wishes to "make him happy."

It turns out that from my studies and those of doctors I've read, the frontal brain lobe can be impaired by too much sugar. Not everyone is the same. In the case of this client, I asked if sugar could be a contributing cause to his depression. He nodded and agreed to cut back on sugar, sodas and sweets. Within a year of improved diet, proper vitamin/mineral supplementation, and a simple exercise regime, the man felt less depressed and noticed a definite improvement in his vitality and concept about himself. He decided to go for a colonic, join a gym, and began to socialize more. He found a woman to date and the happiness he had never known.

Sugar is a drug that we and media-hype keep endlessly feeding our children. Diabetes is occurring among pre-teens. We must also take a look at the obesity in our youth, resulting in part from sedentary lifestyles, a diet of fast foods, and sodas. Food is not a substitute for love.

Take time to involve the minds of your children in wholesome activities. Play together, listen and learn together. Do nutritional research for yourself. Don't expect your doctor to know everything about your particular blood type or body type. There are books on both.

I was shocked when my sister turned out to be AB blood type and I am an O. I had no idea we were so different. For me, wheat is not helpful in my diet, but for her, a vegetarian diet with gluten is beneficial. Husbands and wives beware! He may do better with fish; she with a small steak. Check out the information that's out there. So many people have allergies, and it can often be solved by doing a thorough blood detox and eating according to blood type. Keep the immune system high with antioxidants, and get plenty of rest and relaxation.

Find out which foods will enhance your stamina and help avert heart disease. Don't just bop up with coffee. If you drink a cup a day, you must drink two cups of water, since coffee is a diuretic. It kills the B vitamins, so take it between meals, and not as a chaser to wash down your supplements. Green tea is a good alternative.

At one point I almost died of chronic fatigue, fibromyalgia, and a bad case of depression after a car accident. I subsisted on TV dinners, unable to sleep well or care for myself efficiently. I didn't want folks at work to know. I didn't want to lose clients or to complain. I was trying to take on extra work to pay for another car which gave me little time to prepare vegetables. I ate salads, but on the run with no salad dressing. Quite by fate, I read an article on microwaved food - that it loses its food value with the radiation. All I had been eating was TV dinners! It was a wonder I wasn't dead.

Next, I learned about good fats, a necessity in our diets to transport nutrients to the body. I quickly remedied my diet situation with good fresh foods and proper supplements. I researched sleep aids, and bought a pillow that helped alleviate neck pain. I used 5HTP and valerian root with a cup of camomile tea laced with liquid amino acids and L-carnitine. This soothing drink fed the cells during the night, and I came back stronger and wiser, with a deep desire to help others avert the close call that I had. What a blessing the car accident wasn't fatal, but the lack of nutrition knowledge could have been!

Too many people say, “I don’t need a multivitamin.” The truth of the matter is that foods do not contain the value they did formerly due to soil depletion. In the physical world we are given all that we need, and this now appears in the form of quality food supplements as well as lovely fresh vegetables and fruits. That’s evolution. Men, it isn’t *sissy* to maintain a healthy balance of nutrition. Food supplements are food in a consolidated form that we may well be required to rely on in future. Start now.

It is sad to think that folks would turn to prescribed antidepressants before they would try improving their nutrition with good food, simple herbs, or supplements. A new study finds that antidepressant use doubles the risk of bone fracture. There seems to be a link between depression and bone loss. Fairly new on the market are liquid calcium/magnesium supplements with vitamin D. Check into liquid multivitamins I have, which absorb quickly into the blood stream and are in a fruit juice base. If you have an aversion to pills, the liquids may be for you.

Sometimes with liquid amino acids, depression and fatigue can be avoided. The indications of major depression are: persistent sadness; a feeling of worthlessness, hopelessness, or excessive guilt; inability to take pleasure in things you would usually enjoy; insomnia or oversleeping; dramatic changes in appetite leading to weight loss or gain; extreme difficulty concentrating, remembering, and making decisions; agitation, restlessness, and irritability; headaches, pain, and digestive disorders that don’t respond to treatment; thoughts of death or suicide, or suicide plans or attempts.

We all experience some of these symptoms at times, but you can check your diet to see if a vitamin deficiency may be corrected before you panic. Value your health enough to do this. Undoubtedly you know someone experiencing similar symptoms. You will want to be aware if you are to offer help. Nutritional knowledge is basic to health.

Three aspiring psychiatrists from various colleges were attending their first class on emotional extremes. "Just to establish some parameters," said the professor to the student from the University of Texas, "What is the opposite of joy?" "Sadness," said the student. "And the opposite of depression?" he asked of the young lady from Harvard. "Elation," said she. "And you sir," he said to the young man from Texas A&M, "How about the opposite of woe?" The Aggie replied, "Sir, I believe that would be giddy-up."

Exercise begets fitness and being fit sounds like the happy way to be. Some people would just rather read a book, sit in front of TV or play computer games. They may be quite happy, and this of course, is our quest. But for people in depression let's check out what the major causes are. Billions are now being spent to treat adolescents suffering with this debilitation.

Genetics is a major cause. Psychotherapy focuses on the developmental background of a person. If their lifestyle is sedentary without regular exercise, they are candidates. Irregular work hours such as night shifts interrupting circadian rhythms, and eating patterns can pull down the pituitary gland hormones. Addictions cause depression as do toxic hits, such as mercury, cadmium or arsenic in the blood stream. Lack of proper nutrition can affect the neurotransmitters. Omega threes have been shown to transport nutrients like tryptophan, providing a sense of well being. When someone is in grief, loss, or has complicated social problems and stress, depression can easily set in. Illness, diabetes, or pain pull down the libido. Sugar, as we have mentioned, can also be the depression culprit for those unwittingly craving sweets and chocolate for comfort.

A comprehensive mental health program can help. Yoga, meditation, deep breathing can oxygenate the hypocampus of the brain, freeing up memory loss and constriction. We can draw on inspiring thoughts or music that will implement a change in brain chemistry. People have tried hypnotherapy or visualization with good results. When we line our thoughts up with what is true, we can allay some of the fear and depression. Stay with your spiritual practices.

There are four emotions: fear and anxiety; depression and sadness; frustration and anger; contentment and happiness.

Anger is a reaction stemming from personal hurt. Nothing is hurting you but your self-perpetuating past hurts. Lashing back at another is your way of saying you want them to hurt also. It's abuse and it's a vicious cycle. Anger is the heavy price you pay to further hurt yourself. Stop!

You are an individual of divine origin parented by the Universal Creator. There are no mistakes. Accept that the health and strength you need is within you. You are a unique creation, endowed with rebounding ability. You can bounce back! When you're stressed, float a while. No matter the storm there's always a rainbow waiting.

Then get your buns over to the gym! We laugh with those who joke they don't need to work out. They get enough exercise by jumping to conclusions, running down the government, dodging responsibility, running off at the mouth, throwing their weight around, and pushing their luck. Physical exercise coupled with daily meditation is the best possible regimen to insure good health.

Take your morning walk. Get a swim if you can. Go to your yoga or exercise class. Dance with or without a partner. Take a ball and weights class. The gym offers stairmasters and cardio workouts. The YMCA and Parks and Recreation have programs. Do sports. Play racquetball, basketball or golf. Get moving and feel good playing soccer! Take tap dancing, ballet or Tai Chi.

Recently my cousin sent a news article of her gracious tap teacher passing on. He had taught stars and performers in Las Vegas over the years along with his regular classes. My cousin attributes her limberness and flexibility to years of tap into her seventies. Brain, foot, and hand coordination will keep those dendrites growing. Ballroom dancing is widely popular through our local recreation center. Live bands perform twice a week, and folks come out at 1:30 in the afternoon dressed to the nines. Dancing keeps them healthy and fit; and socializing is a mental health booster.

For playful aerobics bounce on a rebounder, or jump rope for joy. The trampoline effect provides training response for the entire body, including the internal organs.

Your endorphins activated put you in an elevated mood. Runners know they get a high from the regular oxygen input. You will feel so good about yourself, you will never regret the initial effort of getting started. Then don't stop! Exercise every day, and you will live the *happy way.*

However it is to be, is up to me.

Life might not be the party we hoped for; but while we're here we might as well dance. anonymous

Be happy regardless of what your challenges may be.

My Heart Makes Its Own Weather

My heart makes its own weather,
So let the world grow gray;
My heart starts saying April
When April's far away.

In spite of rain and reason
And winter on the wing,
My heart has its own season,
And my heart says it is spring!

Blow wind and bitter weather,
Come care and whistling cold,
An April heart will never
Grow gray or crabbed or old.

Time is a wrinkled treason;
Age is an old untruth.
Heart, keep your changeless season,
Green April, golden youth!

James Dillet Freeman

Stimulate the Intellect

Our chief want in life is somebody who shall make us do what we can.

Ralph Waldo Emerson

True education combines intellect, beauty, goodness, and the greatest of these is goodness.

Helen Keller

To stimulate the intellect one's interest must be piqued. Who can teach someone something they have no interest in learning? The wise teacher approaches the lesson from the student's area of inquisitiveness. If no spark of interest appears to exist, still teaching takes place inevitably by example. Smile, people learn through you! That is why framed on my wall is the plaque that says, "Teach only love, for that is what you are."

People may not be interested in what you have to say, but they will interact by how it feels when they are in your presence. We hope they listen, but that varies with each individual. They will take only what they can absorb, so be prepared to give without judgment, or expectation of measured response. We can't be attached to outcomes.

Our children emulate our actions more than words. Stimulating the intellect starts early in the home, but it's never too late to introduce the concept of culture, music, theater and art. Myriads of concepts can stimulate the intellect. The possibilities are unlimited.

My grandmother invited me over, without my sisters, and proceeded to explain in great detail how she took up the study of china painting from Franz Bischoff when he came to Chicago from Austria. Her sister had opted for finishing school, but Jessie chose art. It was arranged that she would live away from home near Bischoff's studio to take classes. She was only eighteen, but china painting was her dream, and Bischoff was already making a name for himself.

I was eleven years old, and had no concept of Bischoff's fame or my grandmother's expertise. She had been one of Bischoff's foremost protégés, and I flippantly dangled my feet and showed not the faintest appreciation that she wanted me to have her paints, and lessons from her on a regular basis. She said I had the grace and proclivity for art, and held very high hopes for me. All of this fell on deaf ears. I shamefully admit now that I should have been disowned for lack of interest or respect. China painting was something I knew nothing about, though I had seen Grandma's pieces displayed when we visited on Sundays.

Dad had bought us a horse which we kept at a farm not far from the city. I loved riding Taboo and writing poems. I was dreamy and undisciplined, listening to music and dancing ballet in front of the mirror. Regrets are best turned into lessons. Grandma's love engaged my wisdom.

Grandmother's passionate example of producing artistic quality hand painted china taught me well. When I began soloing, writing musical theater, and freelance newspaper articles, I could see how like her I was in my perseverance and perfectionism. Grandma lived ninety eight years without pills or ills. She offered a positive declaration of gratitude every day. She was upbeat, forward thinking and always active. She and Grandpa sang duets. My uncles were in Opera, and musical theater staged for soldiers during the war. My cousins were musicians in Symphony Orchestras.

My father worked in the ship yards, sold Hoover vacuums, and became a honey dealer. He was the least educated, but mother saw to it that we listened to opera, classical music, and gave us ballet and piano lessons. We ate day-old bread so we could afford the lessons. Mother designed and sewed our clothes. We were taken to museums, historical sites, art showings, cultural events, and did nature hiking and outdoor camping.

My parents provided continual outlets to stimulate our minds. We played cards, wrote letters and were encouraged to keep diaries or journals. Quality publications were subscribed to and read in our home. We kept up with current events, and the community social calendar. Church activities found us giving our time and talents. School functions brought out both parents for supportive interaction. I remember my parents heading up a school talent show. My dad and a group of other fathers did the can-can with makeup and ruffled skirts their wives made. If that doesn't sound intellectual, I can assure you, it was stimulating and hilarious. I won't ever forget it!

Mother's family was in the newspaper business, and I would spend summers watching the presses roll while visiting my cousins. That side of the family produced writers and women lawyers.... and tap dancers!

My agile mom did cartwheels on the lawn, and tap danced in the kitchen. She and dad were square dancers, complete with bouffant petticoats, string tie and cowboy boots. What an elegant pair who danced, sang and laughed, who truly enjoyed family, friends, and life.

Everyone deserves to be happy, and mental stimulation plays an important part. Feeding a friend or child's interest with your thoughtful questions, stoking an excited show-and-tell with your skillful observance, drawing out a latent talent into valuable limelight, can make all the difference in another's life. Don't ever think it's unimportant when you listen to a new idea. If something is unfolding there may be many facets. To allow and to witness those facets becoming apparent is a delightful revelation to the other, and to you.

We are magically stimulated as our capabilities are uncovered and understood. Our intellects will sharpen when our ideas are heard, and we recognize that our purpose is taking shape. We want to be happily on track, fulfilling our passions and potential. That feels good.

Helps to stimulate the brain to stay active and lively are: card playing, such as bridge; golf, crossword puzzles, playing an instrument, dance lessons, singing in a choir or chorus and reading the music; tennis, learning a new language or skill. Travel, and itinerary planning are stimulating. Going back to school, preparing and teaching a class or seminar, sharing current books or events discussion, recipe creation, and cooking are just a few ideas. Faith in synchronicity, feeling a part of the flow increases the mental powers of Source connection, and brings joy.

On an air flight a gentleman next to me said he had just spent six hours at the airport. Our plane was four hours late because of weather problems in Chicago. When I queried if it was a business or pleasure trip, he said it was a four day seminar on storage and handling for radioactive materials. He pulled out a thick book and said, "I have to know all these numbers." Then he produced a puzzle book called Sudoku which his daughter had given him before the trip. Numbers are filled in the blanks one through nine; then across and down, vaguely like a crossword puzzle. Sudoku is much easier, though, and I could hardly resist looking over the gentleman's shoulder, mentally adding the right number to each empty square. Games are playful deterrents from fatiguing strain and are relaxing.

Keeping abreast of the latest entrepreneurial ventures could engross the intellectual. How about selling bio-pesticides for organic farming? Davis scientist, Pam Marrone, developed a weedkiller made by microorganisms that live on plants and in the soil. Marrone concentrates natural compounds into products that fight weeds, insects and diseases which will, ideally, cut the cost of growing organic crops.

New concepts are being developed, and we, too, can discover inventive genius as our interest becomes aroused. Don't let yourself become a dullard. Use it or lose it. Read, stay aware, converse and share with others. We could learn alot from crayons. Some are sharp, some are pretty, some are dull. Some have weird names and are different colors, but they all live in the same box!

Writing songs and poems can be stimulating and therapeutic. On turning eighty a few years ago, my uncle wrote his book called *Memoirs of an Octogenarian.* When I read it with tears in my eyes, I made up my mind to also complete my long-planned book. Everyone should write their autobiography. It could be a requirement to cleanse and neatly tie up your past with a bow. Do it for yourself. You are then free to live life in the present moment that you fill with contentment and love.

We must look at the world as it IS, not as we thought it was going to be. That's much too disappointing. NOW IS! Every moment is new. Now is always a good time to stimulate the intellect!

I decided that it was not wisdom that enabled poets to write their poetry, but a kind of instinct or inspiration, such as you find in seers or prophets who deliver all their sublime messages without knowing in the least what they mean. Socrates

Carry excellence within as a mantra, as a presence.

Deborah Ann Smith

I've Learned

I've learned a vital lesson
Worth more than gems or gold;
I've learned from tribulations
To bend, but not to fold.
I've learned to keep on learning,
To exercise my mind
And search for hidden treasures
That beckon me to find.
I've learned to keep on caring
For those I'm prone to flee;
I've learned the art of sharing
With those who turn to me.
I've learned a bit of wisdom
Along life's rocky way,
This simple guide for living;
Be grateful for today.

William Arthur Ward

Be a Nutrition Nut

Be careful about reading health books. You may die of a misprint.

Mark Twain

You must do the thing you think you cannot do.

Eleanor Roosevelt

Have you known someone who is a nut about something? I guess nutrition is a category I'm nuts about. When you teach something you are totally dedicated to, you have the urge to draw others into your consuming passion as if they can't live without it.

Three of my family members died before old age, and I almost did, when lacking in nutrition. I feel so strongly that we must educate ourselves on food supplements, herbs and detox systems, that I'll give to you my web page for the supplements I use and offer: www.victoriamorse.com. Sir Izaac Walton says to value your health next to a good conscience, and I would agree.

Do you ever peer into others' shopping carts while waiting in line? You can get ideas for different meals that way. Once about fifteen years ago I was waiting in line at a health food store and nodded at a spry senior gentleman in front of me. Have you noticed how men alone shop as compared to women? Men go in for just what they need and leave. Most women take time to loiter, reading labels, sniffing out what would suit the family, or their taste buds for dinner.

The elder in line had in his hands two cellophane bags; one with sunflower seeds, the other with flax seeds. As I congratulated him on his choices, he said, "I attribute my good health to adding these and some raisins to my oatmeal every morning." I was so moved by his robust manner and sincerity that I have done likewise ever since.

I grind my flaxseed in a small coffee grinder or the seeds will simply go through the colon without nutrient absorption. Flaxseed combines the qualities of both fiber and omega three fatty acids. Sometimes I don't do the oatmeal each day, but alternate with a smoothie of protein powder, yogurt, fruit, and banana; or a green smoothie with lemon and added fiber. Liquid flaxseed oil may be added to smoothies, and a little L-carnitine, a liquid amino, for energy. To maintain muscle, add glutamine at times.

When you eat small well balanced meals with a little protein, you can increase your metabolism and caloric expenditure, rather than store it as fat. Select proper food combinations. Easy food substitutions are: rye or pumpernickel bread instead of white, oatmeal instead of sugary cereals, chick peas instead of white rice, lentils or butter peas in place of pasta, plain popcorn, not pretzels; sweet potatoes instead of white potatoes, an apple instead of watermelon, strawberries in place of dates, and yogurt instead of ice cream. Include plain yogurt daily if possible.

Fiber, such as oatmeal or All Bran, and beans, help sweep out cholesterol and keep the weight down. Stuck in a *junk food* rut we can go 'round and around without hitting all the nutritional bases until jolted back to attention.

An illustration is the woman who just got off work to face a blizzard with zero visibility. She wondered how she was going to make it home. She remembered a friend's advice that if caught in a blizzard, to wait for a snow plow to come by and follow it. She was patient, and sure enough, a snow plow went by and she started to follow it.

She was feeling relieved and very smug that she had no blizzard problems following the snow plow. After some time passed, she was somewhat surprised when the snow plow stopped and the driver got out and came back to her car, signaling her to roll down her window. The driver wanted to know if she was all right, as she had been following him for a long time. She said that she was fine and told him of the advice she'd received. The driver replied that it was okay with him, she could continue to follow him if she wanted... but he was done with the Wal-Mart parking lot and was going over to Target next.

How often do we listen to advice but use it without proper application? Don't follow along blindly in a dead end pattern. Use sensible variety in your diet. Do the nutritional research for yourself and your particular blood type and body type. Again, there are books and magazines like *Prevention* to answer your questions.

Here is a list of my favorite superfoods: apples, blueberries, brown rice, flaxseed, cranberries, cherries, oat-meal, lemons, salmon, sweet potatoes, spinach, tomatoes, kale, collard greens, chard, walnuts, almonds, sunflower seeds, parsley, garlic, avocados, and super supreme broccoli! CoQ10 and fish oils are vital to the heart.

If an A or AB blood type, choose fish over flaxseed oil, or alternate them. The flaxseed lignans protect against breast cancer by blocking the effects of estrogen. Good oils lower cholesterol and flaxseed shows promise for reversing kidney damage caused by lupus.

The first thing you want to do in starting fresh for optimal health is to detoxify the blood stream and cleanse the colon. My website tells you about a zeolite that traps metals and toxins in the bloodstream and carries them out in the urine. There are no side affects. You may also look up zeolite.com on the internet.

Chem trails in the air, toxics wherever we live and breathe infiltrate the body with poisons and allergens. We can keep the immune system up with appropriate vitamin supplements and antioxidants; and with the zeolite, keep the blood stream cleansed from cadmium, mercury, arsenic, lead, and other harmful chemicals and toxins. Refresh, renew, restore, and replenish your system on a regular basis.

A liquid flush of fresh squeezed lemon in a cup of water is a great start every morning. Without fail, my Dad rose and drank two cups of water before even thinking about breakfast or coffee. A purified system will respond to nutrient absorption more efficiently. You will need to consume less, feel more highly energetic, and most likely find your metabolism infused to burn off fat stores.

For natural control of cholesterol the best zappers are: apple cider vinegar, cranberries, lemons, asparagus, broccoli, cabbage, jicama, cauliflower, cucumbers and most vegetables. Fish, chicken or turkey without the skin are good. If you eat lamb or lean beef, keep the portion size to that of a deck of cards. We do best with a little protein three times a day, and I add a couple of snacks in between, like: ten almonds a day, a cube of cheese, a tablespoon of peanut butter stuffed in a celery stalk, yogurt on a rye crisp, a hard boiled egg, or a turkey slice roll-up.

Don't skip meals. It puts the body in stress mode and actually can cause weight gain. The healthiest thing to do is to eat regular meals to keep the metabolism actively constant, so you burn the calories and fat efficiently rather than storing it as fuel.

You'll find good information in Dr. Peter J. D'Adamo and Catherine Whitney's book, "Eat Right for Your Type." It's been on bookshelves for years, so you can find the foods specifically for your type that will enhance your energy, or those which may be causing allergies and discomfort. Understand food combinations and what acids can do if you don't balance the pH in the system with alkaline foods.

Meat, medications, and coffee are acidic. Most of us run acidic, so we must balance the body chemistry by adding vegetables and grains which are alkaline. MSM is a sulfur alkaline supplement you can buy. Try having salad at the end of the meal to cleanse the palate and digestive system. Eating greens adds mood-elevating folate. Coffee is so highly acidic that it should be eliminated or dramatically cut back if you take medications. Check with your doctor.

The following are some helpful hints about foods: Heal a wound with honey. It kills infections. Use a packet of Fleishmann's yeast for cold sores or herpes. Never drink soda from a can. You will ingest four milligrams of aluminum into your body. Use pear juice for upset stomach; treat ulcers with a spoonful of honey. Fava beans work well for Parkinson's disease. Cherries help prevent gout and cancer. Amaranth, the mother of grains, is a complete protein containing nine amino acids. White corn contains more than double the fiber of yellow. Steam it. Boiling corn destroys the nutritional goodness.

Heft up and sniff a melon. If there's no fragrance, try another. Eat melons soon after cutting or the vitamin C is lost. For heartburn, eat pasta or rice which absorbs acid. Nuts are good for the heart, in small quantities without salt. Higher potassium yields lower blood pressure. Potassium helps flush cholesterol out of the body.

Red grapefruit is best, bursting with limonoids. The healthiest cabbage is Savoy. Buy a pineapple firm; the leaves should be crisp and deep green without yellowed or browned tips. "Gold" pineapple imported from Costa Rica is exceptionally sweet and contains four times the vitamin C. Licorice is good for hot flashes; apricots enhance your love life.

Do you fight temptation for bakery goods? The most weight I ever put on was when I would have coffee and half a donut, or a muffin at work. It just creeps up. I made a rule that if I have a cup of coffee, not to eat with it. Then I drink two cups of water to replace fluids because coffee is a diuretic. You are probably familiar with this story:

After starting a new diet I altered my drive to work to avoid passing my favorite bakery. I accidentally drove by the bakery this morning. As I approached, there in the window were a host of goodies. I felt this was no accident, so I prayed: "If You want me to have any of those delicious goodies, create a parking place for me directly in front of the bakery." Sure enough, on the eighth time around the block, there it was!"

If that's you, don't be embarrassed. That's why you picked up this book! We know diets don't work. We advocate that proper nutrition with supplementation, happy living, and exercise can make the difference. If you want something that works, drop the things that haven't worked, or have sabotaged you in the past.

It's not the food of itself that gives one comfort or makes one happy. Geneen Roth says in her books, "Feeding the Hungry Heart" and "When Food is Love," that we "need to understand the underlying issues of emptiness, control and anxiety that define our eating patterns." We need to silence the "inner critic" to eliminate food and weight obsessions. Obesity disappoints us terribly. We need to find something in the person looking back from the mirror to be proud of! Make a list of your good qualities.

I suggest you find a baby picture of yourself, or one of you at age four, or so. Put it in a frame to place where you will lovingly look at your baby often. Nurture and bless this child, and be the parent for it that you would like it to have. My sister suggested I do this. Our parents were wonderful, but they were so popular and busy with their lives, I often felt very alone.

My picture is where I see it every morning when I awake. I send this child love, and bless the day it was born. I acknowledge that this little person has gifts to fulfill that will serve and bring happiness and well-being to others. I tell her I love her. Face it folks! Nobody else may have told you. You may be all you've got. So tell yourself, "I love you," and then say it again to the mirror.

Start the day doing those things necessary to the health and best interest of the one in the child photo, yourself. I can't express resoundingly enough the wonderful things which have taken place since I have begun to nurture and care for that little one.

Pull out your photo now; value and honor it every day. You will prove that there is nothing more important than cherishing yourself in loving esteem. Miracles will happen if you do! You will find yourself smiling and happy.

Miracles

Miracles, everyone looks for miracles.
We'll find them when we lift up and open
our eyes to see
Love in the hearts of one another,
Peace in the forest, sky and sea,
Joy in the laughter of our children,
Strength in the roots of every tree.

Miracles, open your heart to miracles.
Look within, find the miracle of light
dispelling fear.
You are precious, priceless, worthy;
You have the power to be free;
You have strength from your beginnings,
The roots of life eternally.

Miracles, I'm expecting miracles.
I experience oneness in family unity.
It's a miracle fulfilling my potential.
Miracles are happening as I am willing to see
All things are possible, It's very possible
That deep within I know my miracle - is me!

Victoria Morse

Serve to Succeed

The more completely we give of ourselves,
The more completely the world gives back to us.

The Buddha

We make a living by what we get, but we make a life by what we give.

Winston Churchill

One secret of success in life is for a man to be ready for his opportunity when it comes.

Benjamin Disraeli

My mother used to have some pretty good one-liners, like: "You can't serve two masters, you know." I guess that crisp message was delivered at times when I had homework and wanted to watch TV instead. The word *service* in our family was centered around what was going to happen in church on Sunday, or how we could help in the community or at school. School service was something we heard *big time*, so I decorated for dances, put on the Senior Mothers' Tea, and served as an usher for school events.

My father had a pick-up truck, so he was called into service countless times to help people move, or to transport something for a neighbor. He readily said "yes" with a willing spirit. Sometimes we went along. Serving is fun. You meet people and have a job that makes you feel useful. Visiting the hospital, serving a sick friend or relative makes you stronger. You feel good about yourself that you're there for people.

Actress, activist and mother, Angelina Jolie, said in a magazine article that she grew up seeing her mother live a life of selfless giving. She, too, wants her life to matter. Most of us want to leave a legacy, so I end each of my yoga classes with that statement. "We make a difference!"

Your thoughts and feelings go out to create the atmosphere in your community. Become aware that your service can be merely giving a smile; that your service could be keeping your yard presentable, or being polite and considerate. I know a single man who every year went to a great deal of trouble stringing lights for the holiday season. I asked him if he had family visiting and he said, "No, I just do it for the neighbors." Thinking of others in a kindly way matters, and can add happiness to your game card .

One of my clients said he always mows the neighbor's yard. When I inquired further, he said, "The man doesn't seem to be able to do it himself." Good deeds are being performed silently everywhere. Serving is a way of giving and circulating that gift we know is ours to share.

Dad took the family on a camping trip to Tuolumne Meadows near Yosemite one year. We had planned long in advance, packed for the week, and set out in overcast skies. Always optimistic, Mother and Dad assured us the sun would shine tomorrow. But the sky darkened until all thunder broke loose in a relentless torrential downpour. We had arrived, and dad was shouting directions for each of us to unpack the tent stakes. He had the tarp and three of us doggedly held onto our stakes, soaked to the bone, while he pounded them into the ground. He got us under cover and cared for, and then with big-hearted generosity took his flashlight and waded through rivers of mud to help other weary travelers trying to find camp spots. He waved his light directing cars to safety. He helped people set up their tents and then moved on to help the next. All night he worked for total strangers to safely find places of shelter from the flooding rains.

I remember I was about six, and fell asleep in the car. My older sister related again the details, and she and I cried as we recalled together the heroic kindness and endless energy our father displayed helping others. With each waking thought was the question, "How can I serve today."

When done cheerfully and willingly, your lives are infused with strength of character through service that becomes a lasting example. It was my dad's way to give every *"lady of the house"* a little jar of honey as a hostess gift. "Sweets for the sweet," he would say, proud of his wife, the queen bee, and his daughters, the little honeys. On his passing in the small town where he retired in his seventies, the church was filled to capacity and overflowing at his funeral. We are not remembered by how rich and successful we are, but by how many lives we have touched with love from the heart.

Success teachers abound, and I have most of their books. Elected most likely to succeed, I thought there was something I was obligated to do in life to have received such an honor at High School graduation. In the eighties I studied Arnold Patent's book of universal principles, "You Can Have it All." Stephen Covey came out with "Seven Principles of Highly Effective People" in 1990. Of course I wanted to be one of those, so I bought the book. I had carried around Yogananda's "Laws of Success" and jumped at the chance to purchase Deepak Chopra's, "The Seven Spiritual Laws of Success," a Practical Guide to the Fulfillment of Your Dreams.

I had made the decision my dreams were going to be fulfilled in this lifetime and I was willing to do what it takes for that to happen. Trying to put a time-frame on it, I made one of those mock-up visualization charts, and had to start over when that flopped. Materialistic whims often don't afford happiness. We get what our vibrations put out there, but sometimes it isn't what we wanted afterall.

We do need goals. Without them the mind tends to wander and become distracted from accomplishing anything in life. The Founder of the University of Sedona, Dr. Paul Leon Masters, says, "Establishing and accomplishing your goals leads to happiness and fulfillment. The reason why people have difficulty in accomplishing their goals is because they really don't know their true goals. They are living the fiction of someone else's dream."

If you are living the thoughts and dreams of others and not your own, take steps to return to your soul's purpose, the true purpose intended for you. Surrendering to quiet awareness through your spiritual practices will uncover and re-acquaint you with your original uniqueness and purpose on the planet.

Don't outline how your goals are going to come about! You cannot possibly conceive how the puzzle pieces will fit together, so let go and let God. All we need to do is follow through on our guidance and take the next step as it appears. Your commitment to following through will give you the additional power to accomplish your goals.

I taught a Success Series using the prior information, and more that I learned from reading "The Science of Success," by James Arthur Ray. I also ordered his subsequent book, "Practical Spirituality." You'll find that most successful leaders and teachers devote themselves to one or more spiritual practices.

I asked the class participants to write on a card what they thought success was. One wrote she thought it was synonymous with prosperity, and asked if success can be measured. Is it an attitude as much as tangible money? The others chimed in that it might not always be measured in money, but it certainly could be an attitude.

To be sure, the dictionary definition says success is the gaining of fame, wealth, or rank; the scale or level of gain; a desired outcome or result. To succeed implies the favorable attainment of a desired goal. Another participant read his card which included having meaningful work, a loving relationship, close friends, and financial security. Each read similar ideas about success and we decided we also liked one definition given by Yogananda:

> *Success is measured by the yardstick of happiness,*
> *by your ability to remain in peaceful harmony*
> *with cosmic laws.* Paramahansa Yogananda

We left it up to the class to discover what cosmic laws are, but you get the drift that we must all create our own definition of what success will represent to us in our lives. If to you, it must be a financial achievement, and to another, peace of mind which no one can disturb, or to another, being well-known and popular, what does it matter but to the one defining it? Success starts with an inside attitude of your own worth. You create it.

Write down your definition. Be specific as to what your goal of success is to be for you, and make it something within your personal reach. It's okay to dream big, but it is also wise to build small successes, one upon the next. Enjoy yourself along the way, because if your work isn't bringing some measure of purposefulness, or meeting a need for you to grow, then it can't be the right work for you. In choosing your career, look for a job that you would do for free if life afforded you the opportunity.

Your Will is the dynamo. Never let fatigue, depression, or worthlessness kill your spirit to succeed. Nearly every successful person has suffered a failure, or a series of failures like I have. I've wanted to throw myself into the river, but always picked myself up again. Some sign, some little bird song, a message on the radio, or a phone call will help you rebound. Giving up human sense for the *Divine* is the only way I have known to lift myself back up. Provide some service for another worse off than yourself.

A neighbor in my complex I don't know well, was passing nearby the recreation room, obviously looking for me as I parked my car. She had in her hands a white notebook which she presented to me. "I thought you might want this. You are interested in nutrition and I have collected and saved these newsletters," she said.

I had just come from the library searching out the final authors I needed to complete my Masters' Thesis bibliography. The notebook handed to me contained three years of chronologically indexed material by an eminent British nutritionist. I would never have found this valuable material in the library, and it was just what was required to complete my fifteen-book bibliography!

It wasn't so much the material I was gifted, as I already had most of my thesis completed. It was the genuine desire on the part of this person who followed through on her inclination. That was the sign I needed to take hold and finish the task I had been given to do. I sailed! The words took shape and the ideas flowed from then on. I recalled one day in the laundry room, I had listened and given a personal uplift to this woman who is the care-giver for an invalid husband. She had so desperately needed the show of loving support that day, and in return four years later, placed in my hands the notebook that would benefit me more than any other gift could have done.

We know when angels attend and when synchronicity flows. We feel the mighty power of a good deed making its mark. There is another lady I'll never forget, and I knew her only about a month. It was near Christmas about 1982, and I was working out at New Helvetia at the low income housing center. Excess food was brought in periodically by the Senior Gleaners, and one of my tasks was to leave my office next door and monitor the line as residents picked up the food. I got to know a few people, and this sweet older lady was among them.

She couldn't wait to see me one day, holding a small wrapped gift she urged on me as "a little something for Christmas." I was totally touched. These people had little money, and for her to want to give me something warmed my heart. I accepted the gift and said I would open it on Christmas. I touched her shoulder and told her I would always remember her and her thoughtful gesture. She waited until I finished, and looked at my eyes. Satisfied, she left.

I learned she died three days later. I tearfully opened the gift and it was an embroidered satin cloth money holder. It probably cost only a dollar, but I cried, and told this relative stranger from my heart, that I cared deeply about her and I would never forget her or her gift. That was what she had wanted. She may not have had relatives. How hard is it to remember people with love? That's really what we all want, to be well thought of and remembered because we made a difference in some way.

Success is different things to different people. That's how it will always be. Everything is relative. You can live rich and have big bills, or you can live small and have small bills. You decide how to live a quality life with what you have. Consider this analogy: Life is like a cup of delicious coffee. Your job, money, and position in society are the cups. The cups are just tools to hold and contain life. The type of cup one has does not define or change the quality of life a person lives.

It doesn't matter what size house you have, or what kind of car you drive. Your success is defined by you, and you alone. Sometimes by concentrating on the externals, like how big or expensive is the coffee cup? we fail to enjoy it's contents.

Enjoy your life like you would the finest coffee. Take time and savor it. The happiest people don't always have the biggest or the most expensive of something. They appreciate and make the best of what they do have!

Simply Happy

Everything is simply happy.
Trees are happy for no reason;
they are not going to become prime ministers
or presidents and they are not going to become rich
and they will never have any bank balance.
Look at the flowers - for no reason. It is simply
unbelievable how happy flowers are.

Rumi

Success

To laugh often and love much;
To win the respect of intelligent people
and the affection of children;
To earn the approbation of honest critics
and endure the betrayal of false friends;
To appreciate beauty;
To find the best in others;
To leave the world a bit better,
whether by a healthy child,
a redeemed social condition,
or a job well done;
To have played and worked with enthusiasm
and sung with exultation;
To know even one life has breathed easier
because you have lived-

This is to have succeeded.

Ralph Waldo Emerson

***Smart** goals -* ***S**pecific*
***M**easurable*
***A**ttainable*
***R**ealistic*
***T**imebound*

Cause and Effect

Every action generates a force of energy
that returns to us in like kind. . .
what we sow is what we reap.

And when we choose actions that bring
happiness and success to others,
the fruit of our karma is happiness and success.

Deepak Chopra

Detachment

In detachment lies the wisdom of uncertainty . . .
in the wisdom of uncertainty lies the freedom
from our past, from the known,
which is the prison of past conditioning.

And in our willingness to step into the
unknown, the field of all possibilities,
we surrender ourselves to the creative mind
that orchestrates the dance of the universe.

Deepak Chopra

Give Thanks

All is a miracle. The stupendous order of nature, the revolution of a hundred of million of worlds round a million of stars, the activity of light, the life of all animals, all are grand and perpetual miracles.

Voltaire

He who receives a benefit should never forget it; he who bestows one should never remember it.

Pierre Charron

There are people you need to thank. Maybe your parents are long gone; maybe a relative or friend, or your beloved pet has left this world. Sometimes we didn't tell them everything we wanted to at the time. Did you say "I love you?" If you didn't, there's always the present moment now. It's never too late to say "thank you" to those who have blessed you, or to mentally send your appreciation when face to face is no longer possible.

My teachers I regard highly, and I continue to keep in touch with about eight or ten of them. I would not have my profession without those dedicated souls who had faith in my ability, who encouraged my attempts until I became confident and proficient in my own prowess.

Almost everyone with whom we interact teaches us in some way. We can be genuinely grateful even if the contact is not always pleasant. Holding to gratitude opens us up to receiving more. Just thank them mentally and move on if the energy does not allow you to commingle. Living in non-attachment without judgment will free you to circulate among those like minds with whom you can partner to mutual benefit. We are energy fields of *like* attracting *like.* You will find people moving into the sphere of your consciousness at the level where your thinking and aspirations reside.

I met my primary yoga teacher in a very interesting and synchronistic way. In my gym I was acquainted with the early morning crowd, two friends of which had just returned from Laughlin, Nevada. The couple insisted I needed a vacation and should go. They said the river-walk was lovely and that I would rest and enjoy it.

The next month I flew to Laughlin for three days. On arrival I noticed two lovely people practicing yoga on the lawn. After getting settled in my room, I returned, and the woman and man invited me to join them, which I did daily during my stay there. I seemed to recognize the movements, and they could see I was experienced in ballet, easily adapting to the yoga routines. Discussing our backgrounds, I learned that Mary Frances Edwards had taken yoga classes from Juliu Horvath, who had defected from the Romanian Ballet to dance in the United States in the seventies. He taught Mary Frances in Florida and then returned to New York to dance.

When I returned home I discovered that the owner of the dance school where I had worked, my teacher for three years, had also taken classes from Juliu either in Florida or New York, I didn't know which. I had recognized the same moves with Mary Frances, and realized my ballet teacher was giving yoga prep as warm up for his ballet and jazz classes . My meeting with Mary Frances was significantly pre-ordained. Her yoga video was released and I was the first to purchase it. We have stayed in contact for twelve years and she, beautiful and ageless, moved from Florida to Las Vegas, where we visit together occasionally.

Can I help but be in constant gratitude for gifts my teachers have bestowed on me? Other stories come to mind, but I would like to mention Oprah Winfrey. She has said many times publicly that one of her secrets to success is giving thanks. Billy Graham complimented Oprah when on her show he said about her, "You have made people all over this country aware of the power of being grateful." Billy Graham also said he was most thankful for "salvation given to us in Jesus Christ." Find and establish thanks daily for what evokes in you the most gratitude.

A husband and wife came for counseling after 15 years of marriage. When asked what the problem was, the wife went into a passionate, painful tirade listing every problem they had ever had in the 15 years they had been married. She went on and on and on; neglect, lack of intimacy, emptiness, loneliness, feeling unloved and unlovable, an entire laundry list of un-met needs she had endured over the course of their marriage.

Finally, after allowing this to go on for a sufficient length of time, the therapist got up, walked around the desk and, after asking the wife to stand, embraced and kissed her passionately.

The woman shut up and quietly sat down as though in a daze. The therapist turned to the husband and said, "This is what your wife needs at least three time a week. Can you do this?" The husband thought for a moment and replied, "Well, I can drop her off here on Mondays and Wednesdays, but on Fridays, I golf."

When asked his secret of love, "Being married fifty-four years to the same person" was Graham's answer. "Ruth and I are happily incompatible." Graham said. Our differences are what keep things vital. How much more comfortable we would live if we could be grateful for happy incompatibility. It's your choice to be happy, regardless.

If you must disagree, agree to do so amicably, and make what sets us apart an occasion to compliment another. Be big enough to allow another to express, and small enough to realize that you, too, are still growing. I love a verse of this old hymn. I don't know who wrote it. I just memorized it when I was growing up:

Our gratitude is riches, complaint is poverty,
Our trials bloom in blessings; they test our constancy.
Oh, light from joy is minted, an everlasting gold;
True gladness is the treasure
that grateful hearts will hold.

A dear sister gave me a 3 x 5 card that says, "Thank You for Everything! I have no complaint whatsoever!" She also urged me to "Stay believing in the spiritual essence of who you are." She reminded me of the three "A" words: become *Aware, Accept,* and *Actualize.* Gratitude is a magnetic force which accentuates your appreciation for what is already there. *There is no need ever to envy or to diminish another.*

This story is called Red Marbles. I was at the corner grocery store buying some early potatoes. I noticed a small boy, delicate of bone and feature, ragged but clean, hungrily apprising a basket of freshly picked green peas. I paid for my potatoes but was also drawn to the display of fresh green peas. I am a pushover for creamed peas and new potatoes. Pondering the peas, I couldn't help overhearing the conversation between Mr. Miller (the store owner) and the ragged boy next to me.

"Hello Barry, how are you today?" "H'lo, Mr. Miller, Fine, thank ya. Jus' admirin' them peas. They sure look good." "They are good, Barry. How's you Ma?" "Fine, Gittin' stronger alla' time." "Good. Anything I can help you with?" "No, Sir. Jus' admirin' them peas." "Would you like to take some home?" asked Mr. Miller. "No, Sir. Got nuthin' to pay for 'em with." "Well, what have you to trade me for some of those peas?"

"All I got's my prize marble here." "Is that right? Let me see it," said Miller. "Here 'tis. She's a dandy." "I can see that. Hmmmmm, only thing is, this one is blue and I sort of go for red. Do you have a red one like this at home?" the store owner asked. "Not 'zackley but almost." "Tell you what. Take this sack of peas home with you and next trip this way let me look at that red marble," Mr. Miller told the boy. "Sure will. Thanks, Mr. Miller."

Mrs. Miller, who had been standing nearby, came over to help me. With a smile she said, "There are two other boys like him in our community. All three are in very poor circumstances. Jim just loves to bargain with them for peas, apples, tomatoes, or whatever. When they come back with their red marbles, and they always do, he decides he doesn't like red after all and he sends them home with a bag of produce for a green marble or an orange one, when they come on their next trip to the store."

I left the store smiling to myself, impressed with this man. A short time later I moved to Colorado, but I never forgot the story of this man, the boys, and their bartering for marbles.

Several years went by, each more rapid than the previous one. Just recently I had occasion to visit some old friends in the Idaho community and while I was there learned that Mr. Miller had died. They were having his visitation that evening, and knowing my friends wanted to go, I agreed to accompany them. Upon arrival at the mortuary we fell into line to meet the relatives of the deceased and to offer whatever words of comfort we could.

Ahead of us in line were three young men. One was in an army uniform and the other two wore nice haircuts, dark suits and white shirts... all very professional looking. They approached Mrs. Miller, standing composed and smiling by her husband's casket. Each of the young men hugged her, kissed her on the cheek, spoke briefly with her and moved on to the casket.

Her misty light blue eyes followed them as, one by one, each young man stopped briefly and placed his own warm hand over the cold pale hand in the casket. Each left the mortuary awkwardly, wiping his eyes.

Our turn came to meet Mrs. Miller. I told her who I was and reminded her of the story from those many years ago and what she had told me about her husband's bartering for marbles. With her eyes glistening, she took my hand and led me to the casket.

"Those three young men who just left were the boys told you about. They just told me how they appreciated the things Jim "traded" them. Now, at last, when Jim could not change his mind about color or size...they came to pay their debt."

We've never had a great deal of the wealth of this world," she confided, "but right now, Jim would consider himself the richest man in Idaho." With loving gentleness she lifted the lifeless fingers of her deceased husband. Resting underneath were three exquisitely shiny red marbles.

We will not be remembered by our words, but by our kind deeds. Life is not measured by the breaths we take, but by the moments that take our breath. Remember to make that call, send that card; give time to a child, a pet, or just to chat with a neighbor. Gratitude rewards you richly. Give thanks for life.

Happiness consists of being and doing good.

Mary Baker Eddy

Give Thanks for Friends

If I could catch a rainbow
I would do it just for you,
And share with you its beauty
On the days you're feeling blue.

If I could build a mountain
You could call your very own;
A place to find serenity,
A place to be alone;

If I could take your troubles
I would toss them in the sea,
But all these things I'm finding
Are impossible for me.

I cannot build a mountain
Or catch a rainbow fair,
But let me be what I know best,
A friend who's always there.

anonymous

For Giving

Be for giving.

Giving is living.

Crying is dying.

Live for "now," the present way.

Let go the ashes of yesterday.

Victoria Morse

Forgive

We forgive principally for our own sake, so that we may cease to bear the burden of rancour.

Buddha

Nature knows no indecencies; man invents them.

Mark Twain

Forgive and you will be forgiven. Easy to say, but when the sting of hurt is biting, it's time to call on patience, empathy, forbearance. Put yourself in the other's shoes. See what caused the flare-up to occur. All events and conditions arise for our edification. There is something to understand and learn so that the incident can be turned into a blessing.

I was a college student living in an apartment where a large number of foreign students resided. My daily habit was to sunbathe and swim for a half hour before classes. I wore a modest swimsuit, did not speak to others due to a tight schedule, and generally was focused on my studies.

One day after I had locked the door returning from my swim, there was a knock. Midday, I opened the door to find an older foreign student holding out a bag of peaches to me. I politely refused, and he barged his way into the room locking the door behind him. Fortunately, I had presence of mind to look him in the eyes and say, "Leave, or you will be ruined." I didn't flinch. He obeyed.

There is a power to forgiveness that is like no other. I knew this person was lonely for home, and this was not the way to find his solace. That was it! Forgiveness is not just saying you're sorry. It's finding the truth instead of the falsehood about the situation that sets you free. I didn't have to go find the man and tell him I forgave him. I learned something very valuable. That is, I must never deviate from integrity, stand principled in it, and that will be my shield and protection.

For a short time I lived near the Griffith Park area of Los Angeles to work at CBS-TV. Though I had been raised in Southern California, moving back to the hustling city from Sacramento daunted me with doubts about making the right decision. After a divorce I interviewed and got the job, but felt ill-equipped going back into the work force after being a stay-at-home parent and writer.

The universe has its way of catapulting us out of complacency, so daringly, I had hired a moving van and followed with intrepidation for six hours until we reached Los Feliz Village Apartments. I requested the key to my second floor apartment, and went back to the Spanish-speaking driver to present him an already prepared check with the specified amount agreed to by the company before the trip.

He took one look at it, crossed his arms over his chest, planted his feet, and said in broken English, "This isn't enough." His jaw was set and he fairly glared. I had scraped together everything I had to facilitate this major maneuver in my life. My job was to start Monday, and I had under twenty dollars in my purse. My bank account was empty, and I stared back in defiance. "That amount was our agreement. You unload this truck right now!"

If you've ever seen stubborn, here it was. My hands still on my hips, the man turned, walked back and got into the truck, and drove off. I spent the week-end sleeping on the floor wondering if I was ever going to see my furniture again. Times like this, you know you can live without *things*. Still, the greater lesson was to trust, and humbly appreciate the man who had packed and driven the truck to its destination.

Our communication problem was solved when my sister wired the required additional dollar amount. I learned too, that men of any culture do not appreciate a woman with hands on her hips saying, "You do this right now!" Even though I was exhausted, frustrated, and scared, there are more gracious ways of speaking and acting. The universe nudges us gently to coerce us via life's encounters to find the better way. We create our lessons and experiences. I had to forgive myself my failings, and focus on the job at hand.

More times than I can count, I've been required to forgive myself and others for foibles of the flesh. I stood and watched as we all said our goodbyes after Mothers' Day dinner at my son's. The other mother-in-law, smiling and waving farewell, put her car in gear and backed right into my car. Six witnesses were incredulous! I bit my lip, threw out my arms and hugged her through her prolific apologies. I said, "It's only a car."

That time I got points, but I sure didn't the day it was my birthday. We had birthday cake that night and I was talking to the young men at the table about their school. They boasted they could buy coffee in high school, and the junior high had a catering truck where some of the kids could buy it. Ms. Nutrition Nut that I am, I expounded, after a glass of wine, on the problems of giving coffee to youth. My son rose from the table, said this was irrelevant, and said, "Come on, boys." I was left in mid-sentence feeling pretty stupid, old, unappreciated, and irrelevant.

It was my birthday, so I stood up and proceeded to tell off this handsome young man that I had raised, obviously not to respect his mother. I don't know if it was the hands on the hips thing again, but he hasn't spoken to me in three years. I didn't swear. I said he was rude, and I think I spoke pretty true. I do remember that I had watched him drink three glasses of wine that evening. I no longer imbibe wine. It causes loose tongues and people to say and do things they don't mean.

It was late, I was tired from driving to get there. By every means I implored my son's forgiveness. Overworked, and trying to relate to the boys, I was a dismal failure. I was so hurt by my son's action, cutting me off, taking my audience in one of the few opportunities I had to share in discussion with them. I told him so. When we hurt, we want the other to hurt, and this is the point where we must stop. I was truly sorry, but there was no way to take it back. The Dalai Lama says, "Don't let a little dispute injure a great relationship." Accept that some days you're the pigeon, and some days you're the statue.

I can only forgive myself for standing up for myself, but there may have been a more delicate way. Maybe not. Maybe this man needed to hear it. There are reasons for every event. That's the price I paid to tell what I thought was truth. You choose. It's really not worth divisions in your family. I'm not too proud to admit I'm not perfect either, but lack of forgiveness harms most the one who won't relent. Forgive, and set yourself free. Blame it on the wine and move on.

Time heals almost everything. Yield, bend, and allow with resilience. This is not to say compromise your values. It is to say, forgive everyone everything ...seventy times seven!

I was in Yosemite alone on a little respite. Walking out toward the falls I hesitated at a fork in the trail. A man behind me said, "I work here. I'll show you the way to the falls." I followed agreeably and soon we were climbing quite some height. Enjoying the scenic beauty for over an hour, it suddenly occurred to me we were quite alone. The man had fallen behind me, but I could hear his boots scuffing in steady rhythm.

A slightly uneasy feeling came over me. I looked down, and there my watch had come unclasped from my wrist and dropped to the dirt. My watch had never before come unclasped, so instantly I knew it was time to return. I bent down to pick up the watch just as the guy dived toward me. Alerted, I dodged and laughed hysterically as he plopped to the ground. He muttered something like, "I guess you aren't in the mood." I reached for his hand to pull him up and said, "You big red-blooded brute! We've got to get on back down the mountain now."

Presence of mind gave me those words, and it broke the sinister spell. As we started down the mountain together, he treated me as if I were an angel, and told me much about his life. It was truly a memorable day which happened over twenty years ago. I was escorted to my lodge and felt more certain of the power of forgiveness than ever. Best is when we can get to the pinnacle where there is nothing to forgive.

Let us be slow to judge, merciful, patient, and quick to forgive. We may have been wronged, or we can look at it as a lesson in divine order helping us to clear blockages from a past life. If we take a higher level view, we can by-pass conflict, choose not to attack, insult, or criticize the beliefs of others. With forgiveness we can disregard the illusion of dysfunctional relationships, as what we focus on becomes our reality. Forgive so that you can focus on joy. Happy living shines through radiantly when the baggage of unforgiveness is dissolved.

Reject your sense of injury
And the injury itself disappears.
Marcus Aurelius

Forgiveness is the final form of love.
Reinhold Niehuhr

I have but one aim and one ambition...

Father Mother Good, lovingly

Thee I seek.

Patient, meek

In the way Thou hast,

Be it slow or fast...

Up to Thee.

Mary Baker Eddy

I shall be satisfied, when I awake,
With Thy likeness.

Psalms 17: 15

Foster Feng Shui

Youth is happy because it has the capacity to see beauty. Anyone who keeps the ability to see beauty never grows old.

Franz Kafka

Where would our divine freedom be if external nature protected us like helpless children, led by the hand? No, external nature must deny us everything so that the happiness we achieve is wholly our own independent creation.

Rudolf Steiner

One of my clients came into the office and declared, taking a quick perusal and shaking her head, "This office has no feng shui, Victoria." "Look," she said, "Your *wealth* corner has a copy machine. We've got to fix this." She explained that feng shui has to do with the flow of energy. When the home, office or workspace is arranged so that the energy can best flow for our good use, we receive enhanced vitality. The idea is to create a happy feeling of being at one with our surroundings.

Terri told me she was moving, and would bring over a shelf which I should place over the commode with some plants on it. This, to break the starkness and deflect the loss of energy with water going down the drain. Next she told me I must have satin or velvet in the *wealth* corner, so I bought a gold lamp to sit on a lovely satin runner and

I placed some crystal figurines. I made other changes she suggested, like putting peacock feathers in a basket, and hanging a small mirrored pendant in a stagnant energy place.

I saw rapid results when in just two weeks my income doubled. The freed flow of energy had enlivened my office vibrations. I felt happier, and so did the clients. Feng shui, according to the Taoist laws of nature, has as its basis the harmony and balance of energy so that it nourishes, supports, and empowers you. Literally translated as wind and water, feng shui is an ancient Chinese art.

Einstein's theory E=MC squared is energy equals mass times the velocity of light squared. We are all energy, folks! Everything is energy. You may not be able to see it, but you can sense and feel it as a lightness and balanced well-being; or, on the other hand, if it is negative and fatiguing.

The theory further states that "Mass is defined by the resistance that a body opposes to its acceleration." A river flows with a current. Traveling with the current you use its energy to take you to your destination. If you go against the flow, you use up your energy fighting the current with little left to accomplish your tasks. Feng shui helps to maximize the energy flow that brings the experiences you desire into effect. The law of attraction draws "like" energy into our lives. It behooves us to keep our homes and office workplaces harmonious and free-flowing because we already know that *like attracts like.*

There are classes, books, and maps which show how to feng shui your home. Each item in your living and work space affects you at both conscious and subconscious levels. Examine everything in your environments to see how you are affected by the items, as well as their placement. Crystals disperse and charge energy with their full-light spectrum. Mirrors open spaces as they bring in light to speed up slow, or stagnant chi.

Here are a few hints to follow for dramatic change:
1. Examine and eliminate clutter. Clutter is representative of the obstacles in your life; it directly affects your mental state. 2. Examine your entry door. Make sure it opens fully. It directly affects your career opportunities and energy flow. 3. Keep the air in your home fresh and clean; it directly affects your lung energy, physical, and mental states. 4. Examine the lighting in your environment; dark rooms and areas directly affect your energy levels and emotional states. 5. Remove your garbage daily; it affects your health and your eliminatory system. 6. Examine and update your electrical wiring; it affects your nervous system and mental state. 7. Examine your plumbing and drainage system for proper flow. Clogged drains affects your cash flow, leaking faucets affect your financial and emotional reserves. 8. Examine the exterior of your environment for any dead or dying plants. Death is ultimate yin energy. It works like a black hole that attracts and disintegrates the energy it encounters. 9. Examine for sharp angles, poison arrows and jagged edges in, or pointing at, your environment. Block or fix the fast chi. It can damage your energy field, creating tension and uneasiness.

The above will give you an idea of the intention behind feng shui being introduced into your home. We don't want to allow our minds to be attracted to evil or despair. Beauty is where our consciousness stays light and happy, and feng shui gives you a bagua map which instructs alignment for creating beauty under each of the following headings: Career, Knowledge, Health, Prosperity, Reputation, Relationship, Creativity, Help and Travel.

When you study and align your energy through feng shui to suit your tastes and desires, you are empowered by nature which can bring about dynamic changes, synchronicities, and magical encounters to your life. This happens through energy vibration and your own intention.

This story called *The Tablecloth*, reported by Pastor Ron Reid, is true. The brand new pastor and his wife, newly assigned to their first ministry to reopen a church in Brooklyn, arrived in early October excited about their opportunities. When they saw their church, it was very run down and needed much work. They set a goal to have everything done in time to have their first service on Christmas Eve.

They worked hard, repairing pews, plastering walls, painting, etc., and on December 18 they were ahead of schedule and just about finished. On December 19 a terrible tempest - a driving rainstorm hit the area and lasted for two days. On the 21st the pastor went over to the church. His heart sank when he saw that the roof had leaked, causing a large area of plaster about 20 feet by 8 feet to fall off the front wall of the sanctuary just behind the pulpit, beginning about head high.

The pastor cleaned up the mess on the floor, and not knowing what else to do but postpone the Christmas Eve service, headed home. On the way he noticed that a local business was having a flea market-type sale for charity so he stopped in. One of the items was a beautiful, handmade, ivory colored crocheted tablecloth with exquisite work, fine colors and a Cross embroidered right in the center. It was just the right size to cover up the hole in the front wall. He bought it, and headed back to the church.

By this time it had started to snow. An older woman running from the opposite direction was trying to catch the bus. She missed it. The pastor invited her to wait in the warm church for the next bus 45 minutes later. She sat in a pew and paid no attention to the pastor while he got a ladder, hangers, etc., to put up the tablecloth as a wall tapestry. The pastor could hardly believe how beautiful it looked and it covered up the entire problem area.

Then he notice the woman walking down the center aisle. Her face was like a sheet. "Pastor," she asked, "where did you get that tablecloth?" The pastor explained. The woman asked him to check the lower right corner to see if the initials, EBG, were crocheted into it there. They were. These were the initials of the woman, and she had made the tablecloth thirty five years before in Austria.

The woman could hardly believe it as the pastor told how he had just gotten the tablecloth. The woman explained that before the war she and her husband were well-to-do in Austria. When the Nazis came, she was forced to leave. Her husband was going to follow her the next week. He was captured, sent to prison and she never saw her husband or her home again.

The pastor wanted to give her the tablecloth, but she made the pastor keep it for the church. The pastor insisted on driving her home; that was the least he could do. She lived on the other side of Staten Island and was only in Brooklyn for the day for a house cleaning job.

What a wonderful service they had on Christmas Eve. The church was almost full. The music and the spirit were great. At the end of the service, the pastor and his wife greeted everyone at the door and many said that they would return. One older man, whom the pastor recognized from the neighborhood, continued to sit in one of the pews and stare. The pastor wondered why he wasn't leaving.

The man asked him where he got the tablecloth on the front wall because it was identical to one that his wife had made years ago when they lived in Austria before the war. How could there be two tablecloths so much alike? He told the pastor how the Nazis came, how he forced his wife to flee for her safety and he was supposed to follow her, but he was arrested and put in a prison. He never saw his wife or his home again all the thirty five years in between.

The pastor asked him if he would allow him to take him for a little ride. They drove to Staten Island and to the same house where the pastor had taken the woman three days earlier. He helped the man climb the three flights of stairs to the woman's apartment, knocked on the door and he saw the greatest Christmas reunion he could ever imagine!

Energy flows where attention goes.

Bringing happiness to others is the ultimate path to joy!

Every day you should reach out and touch
someone.
People love that human touch, holding hands,
a warm hug,
Or just a friendly pat on the back.

A ninety-year-old

Guarantee Grace

We no longer have desires. We no longer have needs. ...This is called "living by Grace."

Joel S. Goldsmith

Chance has never yet satisfied the hope of a suffering people. Action, self-reliance, the vision of self and the future have been the only means by which the oppressed have seen and realized the light of their own freedom.

Marcus Garvey

"When I was born, I was so surprised I didn't talk for a year and a half!" That's a quote from Gracie Allen, comedienne of our grandparents' era who was married to George Burns. Her name was Grace and she kept everyone rolling with laughter. If we weren't so serious - if we took ourselves lightly, we might come closer to understanding grace.

Grace is the pleasing quality of good will. It's a blessing. Be one if you want to see one. You want to be very clear to attract clarity. You want to start looking for the blessing in everything. Look beyond appearances and take time for meditation that allows you to clear your mind. Then identify, and catch yourself when you have worries or something comes up from the past. Consciously release it, neutralize it, and let it go.

Fear is behind our sufferings and problems - a fear we're not good enough, that we are hopeless, that we don't deserve grace, that we're somehow a misfit, that nobody loves us, that we don't have enough, that we will get old, die, and it won't matter to anyone. We were too fat, too thin, too tall, too short, too ugly, and on and on in the human scenario.

That's precisely why we are given grace. We get to drop the human shortcomings and look inward at our spiritual entity. That's where the "good" is. Grace gives us that guarantee. There's something intrinsically good in you! That inner goodness can't be threatened, hurt, violated, harmed, or put upon. Grace assures you when you understand its guarantee, that there will be nothing for you to fear. You can call on your angels when in need.

Once I had a client late on a Saturday and afterward, when I emptied my office trash in the dumpster behind our two story building, I accidentally threw in with the garbage bag my key ring which was around my finger. It was 6:00 p.m. and everyone was gone. I tried to remain calm and called the client back, who hadn't returned home yet to receive the call. I went across the street to a gas station to see if there was someone to help.

Mentally, I concluded I needed a ladder. The dumpster was at least five feet high and I had heard the keys clank at the bottom. There was no way I could climb up without a ladder to get in to retrieve the keys, so I was holding to "presence of mind" and the right help being available. "Calm," I kept thinking, as it was starting to get dark. Who would be home on Saturday evening to help me. Several calls got no answer.

I then spied a truck, an old style telephone truck at the gas station, with two ladders. I had asked for a ladder and proceeded to the truck's driver. The whole thing started to be eerie, because the truck driver wore a gray uniform with no name on it, and, while a handsome man, he looked kind of gray in the light. I blurted out that I needed his ladder because my keys were in the dumpster, and after he finished a phone call saying he would be late, he followed me in the truck across the street behind my building to the dumpster.

He hesitated not one instant, jumped up like a circus acrobat, and disappeared into the dumpster. Just as quickly he jumped out again with uncommon agility. The keys were dangling in his hand. I gratefully took them and offered to pay him. Before I could get to my wallet, without at word, he jumped into the truck, drove around the corner of the building and out of sight. I raced after him, waving some money to thank him. I'm a fast runner, but the truck was gone. It had disappeared into thin air. I ran out to the street and looked both ways. No truck. This angel story made a believer out of me. What I thought I needed was a ladder. He didn't even use it. Grace had prevailed. The divine is so much greater than we can ever imagine! Just believe, and accept it.

Teach by example to your children. If they are kind and obedient, nowadays, they won't be able to get onto a freeway on-ramp. Instead of shaking our heads at the elements of "entitlement," speed, and greed that surface all too often on our highways and in social settings, how nice if we could say, "Your grace moves through every aspect of my life." We best live by the peace attained from another realm through our meditation. In the stillness we can realize Grace and carry it over into our daily activities.

Grace is a constant. It is always there, but you may be unaware until it's time for you to draw on it. There was a woman whose husband had just passed. She was dejected, walking aimlessly in a grocery store when she saw a woman at the meat counter pick up a package of meat. She was nicely dressed in a pale green pantsuit, and saw the woman looking at her. "I'd like to buy this for my husband," the woman in green said, shaking her head, "but with today's prices, I'm not so sure."

Unable to hold back, the woman said, "I just lost my husband two weeks ago. Buy the steaks, and enjoy every moment you have together!" The other woman nodded and placed the meat back in her basket, thanking her newfound friend. When the bereaved woman walked up to the register line, here came her friend smiling broadly handing her three long stemmed yellow roses. "These are for you," she exclaimed. They will know at the cash register they are already paid for."

Imagine a world in which angels stand on every corner! There is kindness and joy wherever you look. Beauty and peace radiate from contented faces you pass each day. Let your outlook be one of grace and you will begin to see the evidence of pleasantries occurring more regularly in your experience.

If we would participate in receiving this perpetual gift, we can acknowledge that we are the arms and legs which bring into realization grace here and now. The hereafter seems a long way off. Isn't now the time for present demonstration? Grace isn't something you're going to develop later if you don't start now. It isn't simply for the feminine gender. Are you waiting for the other guy to smile first, give a greeting, or handshake? For a pleasant world, keep a pleasant countenance.

Carl was a quiet man. He didn't talk much. He would always greet you with a big smile and a firm handshake. Even after living in our neighborhood for over 50 years, no one could really say they knew him very well.

Before his retirement, he took the bus to work each morning. The lone sight of him walking down the street often worried us. He had a slight limp from a bullet wound received in WWII. Watching him, we worried that although he had survived WWII, he may not make it through our changing uptown neighborhood with its ever-increasing random violence, gangs, and drug activity.

When he saw the flyer at our local church asking for volunteers for caring for the gardens behind the minister's residence, he responded in his characteristically unassuming manner. Without fanfare, he just signed up.

He was well into his 87th year when the very thing we had always feared finally happened. He was just finishing his watering for the day when three gang members approached him. Ignoring their attempt to intimidate him, he simply asked, "Would you like a drink from the hose?"

The tallest and toughest-looking of the three said, "Yeah, sure," with a malevolent little smile. As Carl offered the hose to him, the other two grabbed Carl's arm, throwing him down. As the hose snaked crazily over the ground, dousing everything in its way, Carl's assailants stole his retirement watch and his wallet, and then fled.

Carl tried to get himself up, but he had been thrown down on his bad leg. He lay there trying to gather himself as the minister came running to help him. Although the minister had witnessed the attack from his window, he couldn't get there fast enough to stop it.

"Carl, are you okay? Are you hurt?" the minister kept asking as he helped Carl to his feet. Carl just passed a hand over his brow and sighed, shaking his head. "Just some punk kids. I hope they'll wise-up someday."

His wet clothes clung to his slight frame as he bent to pick up the hose. He adjusted the nozzle again and started to water. Confused and a little concerned, the minister asked, "Carl, what are you doing?" "I've got to finish my watering. It's been very dry lately," came the calm reply. Satisfying himself that Carl really was all right, the minister could only marvel. Carl was a man from a different time and place.

A few weeks later the three retuned. Just as before their threat was unchallenged. Carl again offered them a drink from his hose. This time they didn't rob him. They wrenched the hose from his hand and drenched him head to foot in the icy water. When they had finished their humiliation of him, they sauntered off down the street, throwing catcalls and curses, falling over one another laughing at the hilarity of what they had just done. Carl just watched them. Then he turned toward the warmth giving sun, picked up his hose, and went on with his watering.

The summer was quickly fading into fall. Care was doing some tilling when he was startled by the sudden approach of someone behind him. He stumbled and fell into some evergreen branches. As he struggled to regain his footing, he turned to see the tall leader of his summer tormentors reaching down for him. He braced himself for the expected attack. "Don't worry old man, I'm not gonna hurt you this time."

The young man spoke softly, still offering the tattooed and scarred hand to Carl. As he helped Carl get up, the man pulled a crumpled bag from his pocket and handed it to Carl. "What's this?" Carl asked. "It's your stuff," the man explained. "It's your stuff back. Even the money in your wallet." "I don't understand," Carl said. "Why would you help me now?"

The man shifted his feet, seeming embarrassed and ill at ease. "I learned something from you," he said. "I ran with that gang and hurt people like you We picked you because you were old and we knew we could do it. But every time we came and did something to you, instead of yelling and fighting back, you tried to give us a drink.

You didn't hate us for hating you. You kept showing love against our hate." He stopped for a moment. "I couldn't sleep after we stole your stuff, so here it is back." He paused for another awkward moment, not knowing what more there was to say. "That bag's my way of saying thanks for straightening me out, I guess." And with that, he walked off down the street.

Carl looked down at the sack in his hands and gingerly opened it. He took out his retirement watch and put it back on his wrist. Opening his wallet, he checked for his wedding photo. He gazed for a moment at the young bride that still smiled back at him from all those years ago.

He died one cold day after Christmas that winter. Many people attended his funeral in spite of the weather. In particular the minister noticed a tall young man that he didn't know sitting quietly in a distant corner of the church.

The minister spoke of Carl's garden as a lesson in life. In a voice made thick with unshed tears, he said, "Do your best and make your garden as beautiful as you can. We will never forget Carl and his garden."

The following spring another flyer went up. It read: "Person needed to care for Carl's garden." The flyer went unnoticed by the busy parishioners until one day when a knock was heard at the minister's office door. Opening the door, the minister saw a pair of scarred and tattooed hands holding the flyer. "I believe this is my job, if you'll have me," the young man said. The minister recognized him as the same young man who had returned the stolen watch and wallet to Carl.

He knew that Carl's kindness had turned this man's life around. As the minister handed him the keys to the garden shed, he said, "Yes, go take care of Carl's garden and honor him." The man went to work, and over the next several years he tended the flowers and vegetables just as Carl had done.

In that time, he went to college, got married, and became a prominent member of the community. But he never forgot his promise to Carl's memory and kept the garden as beautiful as he thought Carl would have kept it.

One day he approached the new minister and told him that he couldn't care for the garden any longer. He explained with a shy and happy smile, "My wife just had a baby boy last night, and she's bringing him home on Saturday."

"Well, congratulations!" said the minister, as he was handed the garden shed keys. "That's wonderful! What's the baby's name?" "Carl," he replied.

Give us grace for today, feed the famished affections.

Mary Baker Eddy

If you pursue happiness it will elude you. But if you focus on your family, the needs of others, your work, meeting new people, and doing the best you can, happiness will find you.

anonymous

Dr. Deepak Chopra says to become the embodiment of peace consciousness through peace practices:

Being peace
Thinking peace
Feeling peace
Speaking peace
Acting peace
Creating peace
Sharing peace
Celebrating peace

Grace is Free

United as one, the inner voice speaks,
The soul of freedom's unity every heart seeks.
Look up at our country's flag, waving in the breeze.
She says, "You're welcome every one
The Grace of God to please.

Who can place a measure, or a certain price to pay
For gifts of love and brotherhood we share along
the way.
No kindness insignificant for those who writh in pain
Investing in integrity will right the wrongs again.

Appreciate each other, building up, not tearing down
For nothing but the purest heart will ever wear
the crown.
To mud-sling spreading hatred can only bring
dis-ease;
While, to see another's point of view,
The Grace of God will please.

Why must we try to please someone
If it's true that Grace is free?
We owe no one, but to ourselves
To be the best we can be!

Victoria Morse

Receive

Receive! It's true, it's sometimes
hard to do.
If you don't claim acceptance,
Your gifts can't come to you.

Receive with thanks,
It's the nicest way to live...
With a cup that's running over
You'll have that much more to give.

Receive Your Rewards

It is one of the most beautiful compensations of this life that you cannot sincerely try to help another without helping yourself.

Ralph Waldo Emerson

What is done for you - allow it to be done.
What you must do yourself - make sure you do it.

Ibrahim Ibn Al-Khawwas

When we do the best we can, we never know what miracle is wrought in our life, or in the life of another.

Helen Keller

As is my attitude, so is my experience. You've taken responsibility for your speech and actions. You may be asking, "But can I maintain these positive emotions?" Laid out here simply are a collection of ideas which, if practiced consistently, will bring you a measure of satisfaction and contentment. You're already reaping some of the rewards from this reading: pride in following through to the last chapter; and certainly more serenity if you are staying with your spiritual practices. Are you happy yet?

Maybe you still don't have what you want. Are you sure you know what that is? The Dalai Lama says, "Remember that not getting what you want is sometimes a wonderful stroke of luck." Your desire to be happy can be achieved by taking appropriate practical steps daily. It's a mindset.

Adversity is a fact of life. It can't be controlled. What we *can* control is how we react to it. We'll discover the value of darkness, and welcome its presence into our lives. It's always darkest before the dawn. Fresh enlightenment is on its way when we've hit the bottom of the pit. There's nowhere to go but upward toward the light.

What are the rewards of non-attachment? When you don't hold on, the butterfly can fly back and land on your shoulder. Being willing to relax and let go allows for the adjustments to take place which can bring your good to you. Tense withholding is like you trying to control the weather. You can't hold back the tides, or clench tight enough to stop the winds from blowing. Yes, help others make it through fires and floods, just as you would want folks to help haul sand bags for you. But then, there's a certain amount of releasing of responsibility when you've done all that you can do.

Non-attachment doesn't mean to disregard or ignore. It means you listen, love, and let transpire what will without judgment. We may not always understand the reason circumstances come about as they do, but we have drawn them into our existence for a purpose. Opposing forces can cause blockages. They are you - one side of you resisting the other.

When you hear news you don't care for, you can lend kind thoughts which may provide strength for the troubled. Are we becoming numb and heartless because we hear a constant recitation of sadnesses? Being happy is keeping your immune system up, loving yourself and others through their misfortunes. Be a vibrant success without losing your soul! Care deeply, but with non-attachment to outcomes. Tuning out is not a reward. It's a cop-out, unworthy of your consideration. Find it in yourself to look past the surface appearance to the true essence of being. Then leave it.

When considering your love partner, it's good to have independent interests and to respect each other's work or hobbies. The rewards for respect are as great as those for appreciation. Your children, especially, will reward you greatly if you show interest in their unfoldment and treat them as worthy of respect.

I wanted so desperately to make it to my son's graduation in St. Louis. Working for the Housing and Redevelopment Agency, I had to put in almost a year early to get the vacation time off I needed. I saved every penny and planned very carefully. My son had been living with my sister's family in order to attend private school for junior high, and wanted to stay through high school, quite a drain on a single mother's pocketbook.

He had no idea that I lived on soup and one chicken a week, using my student loans to pay for the school, while I worked three jobs full time to finish my college degree. Then I was forced to quickly take the job at the Agency to have dental work done and bring myself back to coherence after a nervous breakdown. I was exhausted from overwork!

Fortunately, I had finished the degree with honors, including masters' course work, but the Agency job was an administrative assistant position, hardly what I expected, having a Bachelor of Arts in Government/International Relations. Also, I had completed course work in the Social Sciences and wrote the thesis for the Masters' degree, but trashed it, believing my work would take me another direction. Later, that proved correct.

On a bright morning in May, I drove the six hours by car to meet with son number one and his new wife to head for St. Louis together. Best laid plans did not include the ex-husband and his wife in caravan. I'm generous, and I get along with people, but this was my only vacation in years! I had expected to drive, but my son insisted I ride in the back seat of his Mustang. It was cramped, the radio in my ear blaring rock guitars, the sun hot, and there was no air conditioning. My "ex" and his young wife had a motor home and the idea was for everybody to go to the Grand Canyon on the way. I had not been consulted and felt about as valued as an excess piece of baggage they had to drag along. There was no changing plans at this point. I was outnumbered and had no voice. I sat in the back seat trying to find the good in the situation, but the tears welled up uncontrollably.

I thought to myself how selfish I was. I wanted so for everyone to have a good time. Son number one was in his glory driving his new wife in the front seat, his mother in the back, and his father in the motor home talking over the CB radio with him. Out on the highway, they began chatting with other truck drivers, having a high time, and I muffed my sobs in a pillow with my head down on the back seat. I didn't want them to know I was unhappy, but I was never so miserable in my life. The pillow was wet with my tears when I heard them decide to meet at a truck stop with two other drivers we had been conversing with. The truck drivers said it was a great place to eat, and my son and "ex" agreed to stop.

I had shorts on; my face was tear stained, so I tried to patch up my eye make-up and smooth my disheveled appearance. I sat up as we parked, brushed my hair and emerged from the back seat. Both truck drivers exclaimed in duo, "Who's that?" I had been hidden from view and the drivers were wide-eyed in disbelief. My son said, "That's my mom," and both drivers invited me to peruse and sit in their air conditioned trucks. We had our meal together, and I agreed to ride in the Peterbuilt to Oklahoma. It was so comfortable and the driver had showed me the lovely music collection he would play on the CD player. It seemed the answer to my prayer.

Of course, I thought we would be driving in consort with my family. The driver asked if I would like to drive. "Sure," I said, and we switched places. I slid into his seat. What a rush! driving a new red Peterbuilt down Route 66 to Oklahoma! My son came on the CB radio, "Hear this, Now hear this! Woman driver in the red Peterbuilt! Stay clear!" I hooted at his lack of trust in my driving skill.

It turned out when we got to Oklahoma, the others had stopped for a side trip. I wanted to reach my sister's in St. Louis and to have a visit with her and my graduating son whom I hadn't seen in over a year. I wanted to be rested and revived for the graduation. It was only two days away. I told this to the Peterbuilt truck driver. He told me he was carrying a load of cherries. Reluctantly, he said he hadn't quite mentioned the cherries were due on the east coast.

He hailed the other driver in the White truck, who had also shared a meal with us. They bargained to stop so I could trade trucks, and the driver of the White would get me to St. Louis. I really had no other choice, and wondered where my son in the Mustang was about now.

The driver of the White eight wheeler was carrying a load of dog food. He wore a black tee shirt, tattoos, and a Harley Davidson hat with matching belt buckle that one associates with motorcycle gangs. I called on "presence of mind" for this one, but he also treated me respectfully, giving me the name "angel" as my CB radio handle. I used the CB, trying to locate son and "ex," but my calls went without answer. We drove straight through and delivered the dog food about 4:00 a.m., at which time I was told to hide in the sleeper. We stopped at a truck stop with showers. We paid for them respectively at the *Ladies* and *Gents* signs, and had a fine breakfast. That's when the tattooed driver told me he had to put me on another truck.

He insisted on buying me a western hat, and then carefully selected another new truck with a young driver who was heading straight for St. Louis. I saw him talking to the young man, gesturing vehemently, convincing the other driver to take me to my destination. The young guy eyed me in my hat, and looked more than a little intimidated. "What did you say to him to get him to take me in his truck?" I asked the tattooed one after saying "thank you." His reply was, "I told him I would *kill* him if he didn't."

For the next hundred miles there was dead silence. The young truck driver looked straight ahead, frightened and unsure at my presence. Finally, I ventured that my son was graduating day after tomorrow and I truly appreciated his dropping me off at the St. Louis truck stop. His stern look softened a bit; but still there was relative silence until I yawned, having slept little in two days. The driver motioned his head for me to nap in the sleeper, and I was out for the duration of the ride. When we arrived at the St. Louis truck stop, there must have been a dozen trucks gassing up. I found a phone, and called my brother-in-law to pick me up, who said, "This doesn't surprise me, you at a truck stop."

Ken came in an open jeep. The young driver left without saying "goodbye" while I was making the call. I was so grateful and relieved to be with family, I didn't mind my hair flapping while holding down the western hat on my head for the entire twenty minute ride. What would my sister think? How would my son react to this brazen way of attending his graduation at private school? Who cares! I was there.

The other entourage arrived the next day, and I was high with exhilaration that the long awaited ceremony was soon to begin. This boy was the jokester of his class. With all of his talents, computerizing the lighting for the water ballet, playing his saxophone, and ignoring his physics homework, we were in wonderment that he was going to graduate.

I sat so tall and proud when he came on the stage, last but not least. We started to cheer in the family corner, and then everyone rose for a standing ovation. This boy, the last of his class at a private school, had tested gifted five years before. I tried every way to put before him scientific projects, historical and cultural outlets. Sending him away was a huge sacrifice of love that I paid for from my student loans while I worked full time.

I wanted him to have the finest education possible. I knew my sister and her husband and two children could provide the family he needed in St. Louis better than a single mother returning to college. They were generous. This boy, who had begged to attend the expensive school, received his wish.

My gift for graduation was small in comparison to what his father brought him, a new camera. I could only afford a little present which I had clutched with me in a paper bag during the entire truck trip. In a carefully wrapped box I had carried a clip-on light for his desk; or he could clip it on the bedstead so he could read in bed. The poem I wrote to accompany the gift included words to the effect that this boy had always lighted up my life.... and everyone's.

Imagine how crestfallen I was when the camera was the only thing that interested him. Never was I able to give the grandiose gifts his father could afford. My years of work at less than half the wages of a man paid for six years at a school where my son could grow up in safety, with love, and integrity. I paid back the student loans. Today, this man manages twenty youth soccer teams. He is a Special Editor for television, the father of four.

I am equally proud of my three children. The rewards of having children greatly surpass the disappointments and difficulties raising them. Take heart, and keep on loving to the end. You receive according to what you put in, and not always from where you have invested your energy. The universe has ways of repaying the slightest good intention and deed. Remember the poem by Kahlil Gibran:

Your children are not your children:
They are the sons and daughters of life's longing for itself.
They come through you but not from you,
And though they are with you yet they belong not to you.

You may give them your love but not your thoughts.
For they have their own thoughts.
You may house their bodies but not their souls,

For their souls dwell in the house of tomorrow,
which you cannot visit, not even in your dreams.
You may strive to be like them,
But seek not to make them like you.
For life goes not backward nor tarries with yesterday.

We've heard past generations laughing at the prediction by Dr. Lee DeForest, that "Man will never reach the moon, regardless of all future scientific advances." Nano-technology now says there will be car tires that need air only once a year. We'll have powerful computers you can wear or fold into your wallet. We will be able to eliminate invasive surgery, since bodies can be monitored and repaired almost totally from within.

For a long time we have known that the body cells renew so that we can have an entirely new system in seven years. If your cells are renewing at a negative energy pattern, you will get more of the same. Keep your body and immune system at optimum efficiency, and your cells will renew at that level, instead of spiraling downhill. Imagine that continuing youth is possible. Rewards for this thinking will lead you to the finest foods, supplements, and technologies.

Both the physical and non-physical are made up of energy and intelligence that vibrates. The difference is the rate of vibration. Early in the eighties, what we remember best from Arnold Patent's book, *You Can Have It All*, is his statement, "What you focus on expands." Your emotion and attention flowing simultaneously, raises or lowers the vibrations that create events in your life.

John Assaraf reiterates in his "Seven Natural Laws That Will Change Your Life," what many writers before him have told us. He says "You can literally transform any part of your reality by changing your thoughts and feelings." Everything happens as it's supposed to, even if it isn't to "your personal taste," he says. We must surrender the ego to the perfection of the universe; and, like John says, "grab the steering wheel of your feelings." Choose positive thoughts, and that which you desire will begin to materialize in your life.

Since the law of attraction holds both ways, if you don't like what you see, with a sense of detachment change your thoughts and feelings. Focus on what you do want, not that which irritates or distresses you. Write down your worries and place them in a "Worry Box" you keep for the purpose of removing worries from your mind. Once a month destroy the entries in the box, or burn its contents if you need to.

We empty out the negatives to fill our cups with the qualities we wish to maintain and share. If we desire to fulfill ourselves, it will be in service to others. "Let your process be as rewarding as your goal," says Alan Cohen. "If it's not fun now, it's not gonna be fun when you get there. And if you never get there, you'll resent all the angst you suffered in trying. So whatever you are doing, enjoy it, or quit it," concludes Cohen.

Laughter heals. Genuine, gut-level laughter exudes from true enjoyment. You must find and do what you love to do. Those musicians and artists who know the rapture of immersion into their art can find a deep satisfaction and fulfillment. One of the rewards for a lifetime spent perfecting and expressing an art or craft is the performing, or sharing of it with others. There are geniuses undiscovered. There are creatives and sports enthusiasts who strive to perfect their ability to gain at-one-ment with their creation or sport. It's our nature to find oneness, and in that process come the rewards.

The well-known clarinetist Artie Shaw said, "Art is something taking place when somebody of great skills loves what he is doing, and works at the absolute top level of his ability. An artist does not do it to please an audience." Shaw continues, "An entertainer, on the other hand, is trying to please an audience. Sometimes he becomes so good, he achieves an artistic position."

I was on my way to receive the rewards of my labor for writing my Doctoral Dissertation. A convention and graduation was to take place, and I was boarding the plane to attend. My luggage was searched because water bottles in my shoulder bag caused the alarm to sound. I had forgotten there were to be no liquids, and my beautiful and expensive liquid moisturizers and gel creams were confiscated. I was horrified I would not have them to prepare for the auspicious occasion of my graduation, and I calculated at least $75 dollars worth of my valuable cosmetics, including my toothpaste, were gone!

How could this happen for my special trip? My unhappiness was overwhelming, and I quickly saw that I must let it go. I repeated over to myself, "Just let it go." "Things aren't important. Your joy is what is important." Oh, it's hard sometimes. I didn't envy the young woman her job who had confiscated the goods. I had cried longingly to keep the small unopened gift set my daughter had given me, and when I put my shoes back on, found the attendant had thrown it back in my bag.

I sat on the plane quietly trying to appreciate her doing her job, rather than berating the airlines, or bemoaning the changing times. I thought of everything I could that inspired joy about this trip. It took the whole flight, but I stopped being disgruntled, and had a memorable and happy time receiving my Ph.D.

A young lady was waiting for her flight in the boarding room of a big airport. As she would need to wait many hours, she decided to buy a book to spend her time. She also bought a packet of cookies. She sat down in an armchair in a VIP room of the airport to rest and read in peace. Beside the armchair where the packet of cookies lay a man sat down in the next seat, opened his magazine and started reading. When she took the first cookie, the man took one also. She felt irritated but said nothing. She just thought, "What a nerve! If I was in the mood, I would punch him for daring."

For each cookie she took, the man took one too. This was infuriating her but she didn't want to cause a scene.

When only one cookie remained, she thought: "Ah, what's this abusive man to do now?" Then, the man, taking the last cookie, divided it into half, giving her one half.

That was too much! She was much too angry now! In a huff, she took her book and her things, and stormed to the boarding place. When she sat down in her seat inside the plane, she looked into purse to take her eyeglasses, and, to her surprise, her packet of cookies was there, untouched, unopened!

She felt so ashamed. She realized that she was wrong. She had forgotten that her cookies were kept in her purse. The man had divided his cookies with her without feeling angered or bitter.... while she had been very angry, thinking that she was dividing her cookies with him. And now there was no time to explain herself... nor to apologize.

The Dalai Lama says, "When you realize you've made a mistake, take immediate action to correct it."

There are four things your cannot recover: the stone... after the throw; the word.... after it's said; the occasion... after the loss; the time... after it's gone.

How you think, and how you feel does matter. See beauty everywhere. Walk in beauty. Receive your rewards! The universe takes place through us.

You are everything to somebody...right now at this very minute. Someone is very proud of you. Someone is thinking of you. Someone cares about you. Someone misses you. Someone wants to talk to you. Someone wants to be with you. Someone hopes you aren't in trouble. Someone is thankful for the support you have provided. Someone wants to hold your hand. Someone hopes everything turns out all right. Someone wants you to be happy.

Someone wants you to find them. Someone is celebrating your successes. Someone wants to give you a gift. Someone thinks you *are* a gift. Someone hopes you are not too cold, or too hot. Someone wants to hug you. Someone loves you.

Someone wants to lavish you with small gifts. Someone admires your strength. Someone is thinking of you and smiling. Someone wants to be your shoulder to cry on. Someone wants to go out with you and have a lot of fun.

Someone thinks the world of you. Someone wants to protect you. Someone would do anything for you. Someone wants to be forgiven. Someone is grateful for your forgiveness. Someone wants to laugh with you about old times. Someone remembers you and wishes you were there. Someone needs to know that your love is unconditional.

Somebody values your advice. Someone wants to tell you how much they care. Someone wants to stay up watching old movies with you. Someone wants to share their dreams with you. Someone wants to hold you in their arms. Someone wants *you* to hold them in your arms. Someone treasures your spirit. Someone wishes they could "stop time" because of you. Someone can't wait to see you. Someone wishes that things didn't have to change.

Someone loves your for who you are. Someone loves the way you make them feel. Someone wants to be with you. Someone hears a song that reminds them of you. Someone wants you to know they are there for you. Someone is glad that you're their friend. Someone wants to be your friend. Someone stayed up all night thinking about you. Someone is alive because of you. Someone is wishing that you would notice them. Someone wants to get to know you better. Someone believes that you are their soul mate.

Someone wants to be near you. Someone misses your guidance and advice. Someone values your guidance and advice. Someone has faith in you. Someone trusts you. Someone needs you to send them this book. Someone needs your support. Someone needs you to have faith in them. Someone needs you to let them be your friend.

If you have achieved mastery of anything, you release concern and the need to control it. You share it with ease. Never doubt, You are loved! If you have found only a smidgen of happiness, or a truckload in this book for happy living, it's all right to cry. You're not alone.

Look to This Day

Listen to the exhortation of the dawn!
Look to this day!
For it is life, the very life of life.
In its brief course lie all the
realities and truths of your existence:
the bliss of growth,
the glory of action,
the splendor of beauty.
For yesterday is but a dream,
And tomorrow is only a vision.
But today, well lived, makes
Every yesterday a dream of happiness and
Every tomorrow a vision of hope.
Look well, therefore, to this day!
Such is the salutation of the dawn.

Kalidasa

ALOHA

A stands for Akahai, kindness expressed with tenderness.
L is for Lokahi, unity expressed with harmony.

O is for Olu'olu, agreeableness expressed with pleasantness.
H is for Ha'aha'a, humility expressed with modesty.
A is for Ahonui, patience and perseverance.

ALOHA is the essence of Being - Pilahi Pakj.

Benediction

Bless our world, our community, our homes with happiness.

"Let the walls echo with the heavenly music of happy hearts.
Let happiness be the order of every day."

Martha Smock

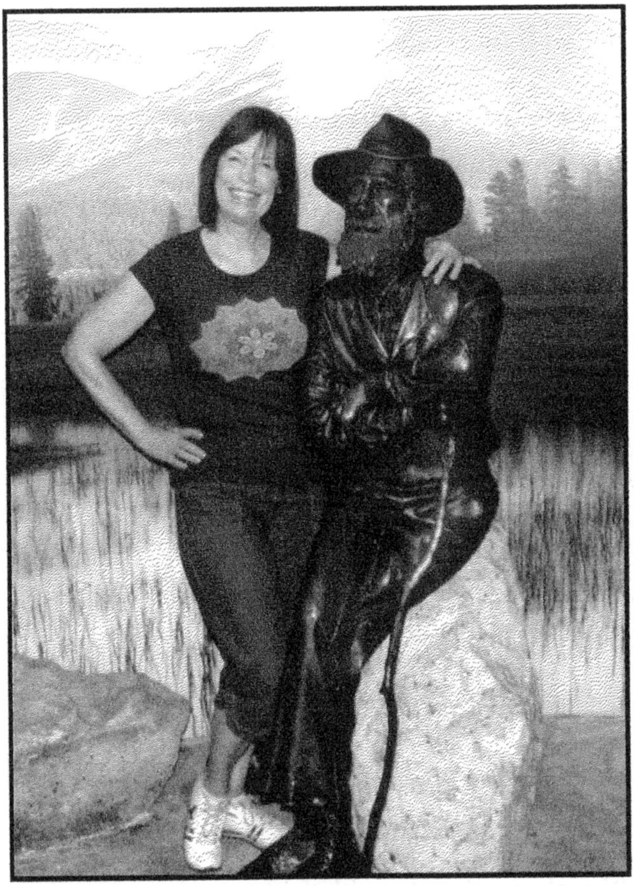

Victoria Morse at Yosemite with statue of John Muir

Everybody needs beauty as well as bread, places to play in and pray in, where nature may heal and give strength to body and soul. John Muir

Photograph by David Foster

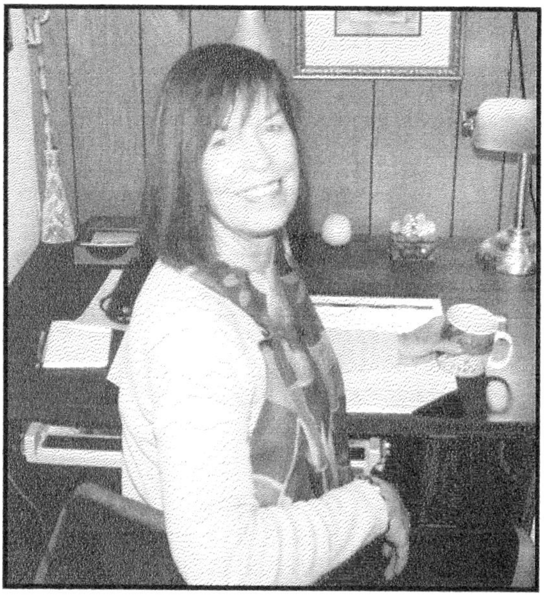

Victoria Morse, Ph.D., received a BA degree in Government/International Relations and a second Bachelor's degree from an accredited college as a non-denominational minister. She holds a Masters' Degree in Metaphysics and earned her Ph.D. in Philosophy.

Dr. Morse is a community college instructor and teaches yoga through the Recreation & Parks District near her home in Sacramento, California.

For seventeen years Dr. Morse saw clients as a health and fitness advisor at her office. She consults now by telephone or email, victoria@victoriamorse.com. She is a freelance writer available for motivational speaking engagements. www.victoriamorse.com

Photograph by David Foster

Order Form

Please send additional copies of *The Handbook for Happy Living.*

Name (please print) ________________________

Street Address ________________________

City/State/Zip ________________________

Daytime Telephone (   ) ________________________

Email ________________________

When you order:	The price is:
1 - 4	$ 14.95 + shipping @ $2 per book
5 - 9	$ 12.00 + shipping @ $2 per book
10 - 99	$ 10.00 + shipping @ $2 per book

Quantity ______ x $ __________ each = $

plus 7.75% sales tax*

______plus shipping and handling**

Total payment enclosed $

*CA residents only

**Delivery by UPS may take 4 weeks

For one book the total w/tax is $18.16. Please send $18

Send check payable to: Light Energy Press
3037 Eastern Avenue, Ste 6
Sacramento, CA 95821
(916) 482-6571
www.victoriamorse.com

Feedback on the book is welcomed to
victoria@victoriamorse.com